THE PROFAST DIET

THE
PROFAST
DIET

BURN FAT AND REVERSE TYPE 2 DIABETES IN ONLY SIX WEEKS!

DR. BRIAN MOWLL

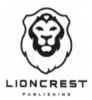

LIONCREST
PUBLISHING

THE PROFAST DIET
Burn Fat and Reverse Type 2 Diabetes in Only Six Weeks

ISBN   978-1-5445-2087-2 *Hardcover*
       978-1-5445-2086-5 *Paperback*
       978-1-5445-2085-8 *Ebook*

This book is dedicated to all of my patients and clients over the years who have struggled with their weight and blood sugar and trusted me to help them along their journey toward optimal health.

CONTENTS

FOREWORD

The human body is an incredible machine. If given the right input, it can do amazing things.

In our years of experience, we have seen many people reverse chronic "incurable" diseases, lose fat weight that seemed impossible, and overcome cravings and feelings of insatiable hunger they struggled with for years.

One of the most common diseases that we see turn around is type-2 diabetes.

Estimates are that almost half a billion people around the world have type-2 diabetes. Countless people are losing limbs and eyesight and dying needlessly every day. But this book is not just for those with diabetes. It's much bigger than that and can benefit anyone who needs to lose fat and improve their blood sugar and metabolic health.

What we love about *The ProFAST Diet*, written by diabetes and metabolic health expert Dr. Brian Mowll, is its focus on "energy toxicity" as the root cause of type-2 diabetes and metabolic dysfunction.

The body can only store so much energy before it runs out of places to put it. Overstuffed fat cells are the central problem in metabolic syndrome, and Dr. Mowll does a great job explaining this phenomenon as he relays how the body works before laying out the diet itself.

It's essential to understand how the personal fat threshold dictates how much we can get over-fat before the cascade of metabolic dysfunction begins, leading to insulin resistance, type-2 diabetes, and other cardiometabolic health problems. Once we understand this, it becomes clear how to reverse the process and heal the body.

The ProFAST diet, as an adaptation of the Protein Sparing Modified Fast (PSMF), is an excellent tool for erasing energy toxicity and helping the body get back into metabolic balance.

As Dr. Mowll describes, the fastest way to reverse type-2 diabetes is to shrink your fat cells and grow your lean muscle. The ProFAST diet is specifically designed to maintain or build lean mass while rapidly shrinking adipose tissues (fat cells). This state gives your body more storage space for glucose while decreasing stored fat and reversing insulin resistance in the adipose tissue.

High-quality protein provides amino acids to maintain and grow muscles. Since protein is preferentially used to build lean mass, the body doesn't want to use it as fuel unless it has no other option. If you are ultra-lean and not eating other fuels, like carbs and fat, the body will be forced to use protein as fuel.

If you have type-2 diabetes, insulin resistance, or metabolic syndrome, your body is typically over-fat, so it will tap those fat stores for fuel when you're in an energy deficit. This increase in fat burning shrinks the fat cells and reduces insulin resistance.

As Dr. Mowll describes in Chapter 2, The ProFAST diet also helps get your hormones in balance and leads to better hunger control. When you follow this plan, gone are the days of afternoon energy crashes or sugar cravings two hours after eating a meal high in carbs and refined sugars.

We have worked with clients and implemented our own version of the PSMF for over fifteen years. Time and time again, clients can't believe how satiated they feel when following this plan, even with days that only include 700 calories! This feeling results from controlling hormones and the hunger that can result from an imbalance in energy.

In *The ProFAST Diet*, we also love how Dr. Mowll keeps the focus on nutrient dense whole foods. We have found that focusing on the most vitamins and minerals per calorie speeds the healing process and improves satiety. The body needs micronutrients to thrive, and getting those from food while limiting caloric energy is the best path to positive and lasting results.

Many people don't realize that animal proteins are some of the most nutrient dense foods you can eat. This benefit is why prioritizing protein naturally helps increase nutrient density.

This approach is potent for reversing metabolic dysfunction. You can rapidly shrink the amount of fat stored in your adipose and thus reverse insulin resistance. We have seen it countless times with clients. One of our clients, Ann, shared this story:

I used to weigh 230 (pounds), and about ten years ago, I dropped to 155, gained some, and have been yo-yo-ing between 200 and 170 for a decade now.

I was doing "lazy" keto often and discovered I had no trouble maintaining while on keto, but I really was often hungry and wasn't losing. Though "lower" carb always helps, I was doing net carbs and probably not really in ketosis a lot of the time.

After years of waffling, she implemented a stricter keto diet of fewer than twenty grams of carbohydrates per day and started losing significant weight. She added our thirty-day cleanse and then started using the PSMF. In three months, she's lost over twenty pounds and is still going!

She told us, "I'm pretty happy where I'm heading! Loving not being hungry; it feels like the struggle is over!"

The ProFAST diet is a powerful tool for rapid fat loss. If you're ready to make some changes to lose weight, improve blood sugar, and regain your metabolic health, dive in and let Dr. Mowll guide you through how it's done in this amazing book.

—CRAIG AND MARIA EMMERICH, INTERNATIONAL BESTSELLING AUTHORS OF *THE PROTEIN SPARING MODIFIED FAST COOKBOOK*

INTRODUCTION

I needed to do something drastic.

I had just woken up with my pillow soaked in sweat and my heart racing. It was about three o'clock in the morning, and I went downstairs, pulled out my blood pressure machine, and hooked myself up. What I saw on the display thoroughly shocked and frightened me. My blood pressure was higher than it had ever been at 190/120. Not only that, but I felt hot, swollen, and sick. It was at that moment that I decided to do something profoundly different.

I felt like I was on a train moving toward a life that I didn't want—one of obesity, diabetes, medications, disease, and early death. If I didn't change right away, I felt that I might never be able to stop the momentum. And I had that sinking feeling in my chest that it was almost too late.

The thing is, I should have known better. I had been practicing for almost ten years, helping people prevent and reverse chronic disease with nutrition and lifestyle management. I had seen the worst of the worst when it comes to diabetes and metabolic problems. I had images etched into my mind of people losing their feet, going blind, injecting insulin, and lying in bed on kidney dialysis because they didn't stop it in time. Still, I had let it happen.

Over the preceding three years, I had slowly gained thirty pounds. It had been a tough period in my life. I got divorced, moved several times, ended a business relationship with another doctor, and had a lot of financial stress. At times, my life seemed out of control. So, I ate. My diet wasn't even that bad except for the popcorn and fries that I enjoyed a bit too often, but I was overeating at night while worrying about my future.

Have you ever felt like you were at a crossroads with your health? Like you had to do something radically different or you might lose your health forever? That's exactly how I felt.

I had heard about the protein-sparing modified fast and had researched it as a potential treatment option for my patients with obesity and diabetes but never thought that I would need it. It was a protein-centric, energy-restricted diet designed to help people maintain and protect lean body mass while losing weight or during illness.

There were dozens of studies showing the effectiveness of this program, but it wasn't easy. I knew that I needed something that would produce rapid results and would work if I committed to it, and I felt confident that the PSMF could provide that type of success. So, that's what I did.

During the next several months, I lost the thirty pounds that I had gained in the three years before that and was able to shed an additional twenty pounds while cutting my body fat by almost

20 percent and adding muscle. More importantly, I was able to normalize my blood sugar, blood pressure, lipids, and hormone levels while creating more energy and feeling better than I ever had. The program completely changed my life.

Since my transformation, I've helped hundreds of my patients and clients using an adapted version of the program that I called my "secret weapon." My clients have lost weight, reversed type-2 diabetes and pre-diabetes, reduced hypertension, eliminated medications, and gained the mental and physical health they desired.

After ten years, working with hundreds of clients, the latest evolution of my secret weapon, now called the ProFAST diet, is outlined in this book.

YOUR OWN TURNING POINT

Let me guess. You're reading this right now because you need to make a significant change as well. Perhaps you're feeling frustrated with your weight or blood sugar levels. Maybe you feel cheated by your doctor because they never do anything to fix the problem and only want to prescribe medication.

You're probably concerned, like I was, about your future and what might happen if you continue on the path that you are on. Maybe you worry about having a heart attack or stroke, losing your eyesight or a limb, or not being able to enjoy your family and retirement because your health is suffering.

If you're like most of my patients and clients, you probably hate the idea of being or becoming diabetic, taking drugs for the rest of your life, and depending on others to take care of you.

Does this describe you?

If so, I wrote this book for you.

Many people feel embarrassed by their weight or diabetes diagnosis and feel guilty about the diet and lifestyle choices that created the situation.

You don't need to feel that way anymore.

This book provides a road map to guide you toward overcoming the challenges that have stopped you in the past. If you follow the steps outlined in *The ProFAST Diet*, you can reach your goals and transform your health, just as I did.

In this program, you can expect to burn fat—lots of it. Most people will lose ten pounds within the first two weeks. They'll drop fifteen to twenty pounds after four weeks and up to thirty pounds after eight. Most people see dramatic improvements in blood sugar levels, blood pressure, and lipids during the ProFAST diet.

You'll probably find that once you get through the first few days of the program, it will be remarkably easy to stick to it. That's because protein, the primary macronutrient in the diet, has the most potent effect on satiety, and the ketones your body is producing will suppress appetite as well.

Also, you'll likely notice an almost immediate improvement in the way that you feel. When you start liberating the stored energy from your fat cells and your body starts burning all that fat, you'll feel full of life and vitality, with a clear mind and a supercharged body.

As you progress through *The ProFAST Diet*, the positive changes will often start to build. As you lose body fat and lower circulating insulin levels, your blood pressure will likely come down, and you'll retain less fluid. With lower blood sugar and lower insulin, you'll reduce your risk of developing diabetes or start to reverse its progression.

Many people also report that they sleep better, have more sexual desire, have a clearer mind and better memory, and have less inflammation. Studies show that with lower weight, body fat, and insulin levels, the risk for many types of cancer reduces dramatically.

There's also a direct link between blood sugar, insulin resistance, and Alzheimer's disease, and as you improve these markers, your risk for dementia can decrease as well.

I've seen these changes happen firsthand in hundreds of my patients and clients over the years, and I know this program can work for you, too.

It's not easy. This program is an aggressive plan designed for people who want to get results quickly and effectively. It's going to take a lot of effort from you, but if you can commit to it, I've seen that it works. And my training as a Certified Diabetes Care and Education Specialist (CDCES), nutritionist, functional medicine physician, and Master Licensed Diabetes Educator (MLDE) has helped me understand why.

Working inside an endocrinology practice, I directly saw the limitations of conventional medicine. I could feel the frustration of our patients as they continued to gain weight and struggle with their blood sugar levels on the traditional diet program recommended by most doctors and dietitians.

Later in my functional medicine practice, I was also able to witness the joy, fulfillment, and delight in my patients who overcame diabetes, lost weight, eliminated medication, and rejuvenated their health.

I've done everything that I outline in this book myself, and I've used it with hundreds of patients and clients as well. Now, I want to help you experience the same thing for yourself. That's what this book and the ProFAST diet are all about.

In simple and engaging terms, I'll share with you the science behind the protein-sparing modified fast. I'll delve into the importance of protein for maintaining and protecting lean body mass and explain the protein-to-energy ratio. I'll discuss how ketones can provide you that unique boost to stay sharp and energized and help you develop a better understanding of diabetes, blood sugar, insulin resistance, and weight-loss dynamics.

In the second section, I'll walk you step by step through the ProFAST diet and explain exactly how to get the best results possible. I'll answer the most common questions about the plan and give you some insider tips and strategies to succeed.

To help you implement the program, I've also included fifty recipes in the back of the book, which you can use to visualize the food included in the ProFAST diet and how to construct healthy and exciting meals.

Like any new program designed to help you lose weight and lower your blood sugar, it's essential to involve your primary care physician in your plan. Discuss your health goals with them, and let them know that you'd like to use the ProFAST diet to improve your health and jump-start your progress. Ask them to help you coordinate your labs and supervise your health through this process to help you succeed with the program.

This program is the beginning of a new journey. It's helped me to lose weight and stay lean, regain normal blood pressure and blood sugar, and handle stress better, knowing that I'm in control of my health.

In just a few months, you could be ready to trade diabetes, high blood sugar, and medications for smaller-sized clothes, more peace of mind, and a healthier future.

I'm excited to share this journey with you, and after you turn the corner, I'd love to hear about your success and transformation as well!

CHAPTER 1

THE TRUTH ABOUT TYPE-2 DIABETES

When I walked into the exam room, Kathy was sitting on the table with tears streaming down her face. She was upset and seemed like she was about to erupt. I looked at her and asked the question that I was trained not to ask: "I can tell you're upset," I said gently. "What's going on?"

For the next fifteen minutes, Kathy shared with me how she was doing everything she was told to do, but nothing was working. Her blood sugar was getting higher. She had gained another six pounds, and she was scared that we were going to make her start taking insulin.

Her fears were justified. As a Certified Diabetes Educator (CDE) in a busy endocrinology practice, my primary job was to make sure patients were taking their medication and avoiding low blood sugar (hypoglycemic) episodes. And the endocrinologist that I was working for—we'll call her Dr. L—had already told me that we'd be starting Kathy on insulin. I was to train her on how to use it that day.

Kathy told me how much her father had suffered on insulin and how she saw that as his first step toward the grave. Kathy had been on a dozen different diets because she'd been told that was the only way to avoid insulin, and she felt like a failure. She was exhausted. She was tired of pricking her fingers, tracking her blood sugar, and trying to figure out what to eat.

The truth is that Kathy was not the failure. We failed her. The system failed her. The conventional diabetes medical machine, with its scores of medications and specialist physicians, was not helping her. It was making her worse.

As I looked at Kathy that day—sitting on my exam table, filled with frustration, fear, and hopelessness—I realized that I needed to change my approach.

I already knew that what we were doing with our patients could be improved, but I was there to get experience and learn from "the best." Instead of learning to take better care of people, I had learned to ignore my gut feeling that something was wrong. I turned my eyes away from the boxes of donuts, bagels, and cookies delivered to the office staff every day. I learned to justify the parade of pharmaceutical reps coming in and out of the office, lining the pockets of Dr. L and the other doctors with exorbitant consulting and speaking fees.

I couldn't do it anymore.

After my shift that day, I left and never went back. I made the decision to start my own practice and find a way to get people like Kathy the help that they desperately needed.

Kathy is not so much the exception but the rule. Diabetes is a wholly misunderstood condition, even among the most highly trained and well-respected physicians, dietitians, and diabetes educators—and that misunderstanding is passed along to their patients every day.

THE MISINFORMED MASSES

According to the Centers for Disease Control and Prevention, more than 34 million Americans have diabetes. Approximately 90–95 percent of those have type-2 diabetes, which is considered a preventable disease.

Years ago, virtually everyone with type-2 diabetes was over the age of forty-five, but in the past decade, more children and young adults are developing it.[1][2] Yet, if you were to ask the millions of people who developed diabetes how they got it, many would shrug, unaware of what was going on inside their bodies. If pressed, a good majority would admit to overeating sugar and processed food over their lifetime or perhaps not getting enough exercise. Most people blame the diabetes epidemic on these two factors alone.

But things rarely are as simple as they seem, and type-2 diabetes is no exception.

Diabetes is *not* the same as high blood sugar.

High blood sugar has a name. It's called hyperglycemia. There are many causes of hyperglycemia, including illness or infection; elevated cortisol from stress, trauma, and chronic pain; certain medications such as steroids and diuretics; and yes, diabetes. In other words, diabetes is one of several causes of hyperglycemia and is not the same as high blood sugar.

Why is this distinction so important? Because every significant treatment approved for diabetes has the primary goal of lowering blood sugar. Diabetes drugs are known as hypoglycemic agents because of their blood-sugar-lowering effect. This fact isn't necessarily bad, except that most physicians use medications as their primary treatment approach, which means that they are only treating a symptom (really, a sign) of diabetes, rather than the problem itself.

In truth, type-2 diabetes is a complex metabolic problem involving many different organs, systems, and hormones, resulting in faulty processing of glucose and fat, which leads to high blood sugar, weight gain, and many other health issues.

High blood sugar is a sign of diabetes, not the cause.

I know that's a lot to unpack, so let's start at the beginning and work our way through this information to fully understand how and why type-2 diabetes develops in the first place.

WHAT IS TYPE-2 DIABETES?

Type-2 diabetes is a condition that occurs when your body is not able to effectively regulate fuel homeostasis, resulting in high blood sugar. Fuel homeostasis describes the various states that occur when you eat food and break it down into usable energy. When food enters the body, certain hormones change, and your organs prepare to metabolize the incoming fuel. Your body burns two primary energy sources: fat (fatty acids) and sugar (glucose). These fuels either directly energize the cells (like in red blood cells), or they enter the mitochondria within the cells to get converted into ATP, which is cellular energy.

In order to get into the cells, these fuels need to go through portals, like doors that are guarded by security. Glucose molecules can only get into the cell with a special key—a hormone called insulin, which I'll discuss more in the next chapter.

In type-1 diabetes, the specialized cells in the pancreas that produce insulin are not functional. Therefore, the pancreas cannot produce enough insulin to handle the glucose in the blood, and without injecting external insulin, blood sugar rises.

Type-2 diabetes is different. In type 2, the pancreas still makes insulin, but the body's cells become resistant to insulin and don't respond appropriately. It's like the lock is jammed—we have the key, but it doesn't work. In both scenarios, the result is high blood sugar levels over extended periods, which leads to health complications such as heart disease and nerve and kidney damage.

Solving type-2 diabetes is not about increasing insulin output (with medications like sulfonylureas) or circulating insulin (through insulin injections). It's about improving the way the cells, particularly in the muscles and liver, respond to insulin to absorb glucose from the blood. This makes insulin resistance the foundational root cause of type-2 diabetes—as well as obesity, metabolic syndrome, Alzheimer's disease, and other metabolic health imbalances.

THE PURPOSE OF INSULIN

To better understand how the hormone insulin works, let's take a look at what happens in the body when you eat a meal.

Once your body has broken down your food into its main components (sugars, amino acids, fatty acids), glucose is absorbed directly through the gut lining, which sends a signal to your pancreas to produce and release insulin. The main job of insulin is to move energy from your bloodstream into your cells to use or store.

Insulin receptors within your cells are similar to other cell receptors—when exposed to too much of a good thing, they eventually become resistant to that very thing. It's called desensitization. Just as we can become desensitized to caffeine, alcohol, the clothes on our back, or noise, the body will become desensitized to insulin after being overexposed.

At first, it takes very little insulin to drive fuel into your cells. But the higher the insulin levels in your blood, the more bathed in insulin the cells become. This leads to the development of resistance as a protective mechanism to the very thing they are supposed to respond to. So your body requires more insulin to do the same job.

Too much insulin leads to insulin resistance, which leads to the production of even more insulin. Meanwhile, another nasty situation is brewing.

Blood sugar, or glucose, is stored in your muscles and liver, and these storage areas only have a limited amount of space. When you're not physically active throughout the day (and don't burn through the sugar stored in your muscles) and eat a constant supply of energy (from carbs and fat), you eventually run out of room for all the glucose.

Once the glucose storage in your liver and muscles is full, all of the extra glucose gets converted into fat and stored in your fat cells. This fat storage leads to weight gain and an expansion of the fat cells under the skin. Eventually, even your fat cells cry, "Uncle!" because they are running out of space.

While fat cells can significantly expand, they have their limits. Once the fat cells are full, they become insulin resistant as well, and the extra glucose gets stored as fat in your muscles and organs such as the liver and pancreas.

When the pancreas becomes clogged with fat, it can no longer produce insulin properly, and insulin levels start to decrease. This reduction in insulin causes even higher blood sugar levels, which eventually leads to type-2 diabetes. That's when the medication merry-go-round begins.

THE OTHER SIDE OF THE EQUATION

Like insulin, glucagon is also a hormone secreted by your pancreas. Insulin is released when your blood sugar starts rising, and glucagon gets secreted when your blood sugar is falling, usually between meals or when exercising. When glucagon sends out a signal, the stored glycogen in your muscles and liver gets broken down into free glucose. Glucagon also tells the fat cells to start releasing fatty acids to be burned for fuel in the cells.

In other words, glucagon increases fat burning.

The majority of people eat way too often and overeat processed and refined sugar and grains like bread, white rice, pasta, and pastries. This overconsumption leads to chronically high insulin levels and low glucagon. That translates to lots of *fat storage* and not much *fat burning*.

When we consume an abundance of dietary carbohydrates, the pancreas is continuously pumping out insulin, which sends the signal to store energy in the form of fat.

When we stop eating or reduce carbohydrate foods, insulin levels start to fall, and glucagon rises, leading to an increase in the metabolism of stored fuels, like glycogen and fat.

In the low-carb scenario, the pancreas continually secretes glucagon, which sends the signal to release stored energy. The first source of energy is sugar stored in the muscles and liver as glycogen. But your body will burn through this stockpile quickly and will need to turn to its long-term energy repository. Since the muscles and organs are considered functional tissue, necessary for survival, the body gets the rest of its energy needs met from stored body fat.

This diet is not as simple as cutting back on calories. It's about what you eat specifically and how it affects the hormones and metabolism in your body. The key to optimizing blood sugar and losing weight is to keep your blood glucose levels balanced so that glucagon can be released and the body can burn stored body fat as fuel.

In other words, weight gain, insulin resistance, and type-2 diabetes are not all about carbohydrates.

Even though it's widely accepted that carbohydrate foods contain sugar and starch (long chains of sugar) and have the most significant impact on insulin and blood sugar levels, type-2 diabetes isn't caused simply by overeating carbs. Instead, type-2 diabetes is the perfect metabolic storm.

According to Dr. Ted Naiman, family medicine physician and

author of *The P:E Diet*, overconsuming energy, no matter what the source (both carbohydrates and fat), along with not being physically active enough to burn the extra fuel, causes "energy toxicity." An overabundance of energy, coupled with insulin resistance caused by various factors such as environmental toxins, stress and cortisol, poor sleep, and inflammation, leads to a dysfunction in fat storage and glucose balance. These factors combine to cause type-2 diabetes as well as most of the complications associated with high blood sugar.

DIAGNOSING THE PROBLEM

Diabetes is diagnosed using blood glucose levels and a test called hemoglobin A1c (HbA1c), measuring a percentage of glycation (sugar-coating) on red blood cell hemoglobin. Normal blood glucose readings are 70–99 mg/dl fasting, below 140 mg/dl after meals, and an HbA1c of 4.0–5.6 percent. If blood sugar is 100–125 mg/dl fasting or HbA1c is 5.7–6.4 percent, it's termed pre-diabetes or glucose intolerance. Once the blood glucose levels are higher than 126 mg/dl or the HbA1c is 6.5 percent or more, you've reached full-blown diabetes.

Again, the big problem with this diagnostic criterion is that it does nothing to identify the root cause of diabetes or explain why the blood sugar is elevated. When high blood sugar is the primary treatment target, even if the treatment is successful, the person still has diabetes because the treatment has ignored the root cause.

Unfortunately, this leads to many people still suffering from devastating diabetes complications, such as blindness, loss of limbs, kidney failure, heart attack, stroke, Alzheimer's disease, and sexual dysfunction, even though they have been treated with diabetes medications.

CAUSE AND EFFECT

Your body needs fuel to function, just like an automobile. Like your car, you need to make sure you put fuel in your tank if you want to keep going.

While fuel is essential for your car engine to work, what happens when you put too much fuel in your car's gas tank? The tank runs out of space, and the gas begins to overflow and run down onto the pavement. If you keep pumping gas, a large puddle will form. If a passing motorist happens to flick their lit cigarette out the window, the puddle of gas will ignite, and the entire gas station will blow sky high.

Admittedly, that's a little dramatic, but the point is that having too much energy spilling out of your cells can lead to nasty consequences.

Initially, this puddling of energy happens in the liver and muscles, with full glycogen depositories leading to an overflow of glucose from these organs. This glucose is converted to fat and stockpiled in the fat cells, where we have much more room for storage.

Once the fat cells are full, however, the body is in real trouble. Now, there is fat overflowing from the adipocytes, and the glucose spilling out of the liver and muscles has nowhere to go. This overflow leads to high circulating glucose and fat (triglycerides) and fat deposition in the organs, such as the liver, heart, and pancreas.

And sugar in particular won't just go away.

Did you ever have one of those friends who, when they had

nothing better to do, would hound you all the time? They call every five minutes to see what you're doing, and when you tell them you're busy, they call you five minutes later to see if you want to do something. That's sugar in your body when it has no place to go and nothing to do.

The sugar that isn't being used for fuel and can't be stored gloms onto the protein structure of cells in a process known as glycation. The result of this process are compounds called *advanced glycation end products*, or AGEs. This acronym works well because AGEs cause your body to break down quickly and age prematurely.

Glycation wreaks havoc on your body. It leads to oxidative stress and chronic inflammation and damages connective tissue and the delicate lining inside the blood vessels, known as the endothelium. The damage caused by glycation, oxidative stress, inflammation, and poor circulation leads to the devastating consequences of diabetes. Let's look at a few of them.

HEART DISEASE

If you have diabetes, according to the American Heart Association, your risk of heart disease is more than twice someone with normal blood sugar. It's not just diabetes, though. Evidence shows that the insulin resistance associated with pre-diabetes and metabolic syndrome also dramatically increases the risk of cardiovascular disease, even with normal blood sugar levels.[3]

High blood glucose levels cause your blood vessels to harden and lose their elasticity. This damage leads to your arteries becoming narrower, restricting blood flow.

The inflammation caused by glycation also damages the lining of your arteries, which causes plaque buildup. This plaque reduces the amount of oxygen-rich blood to your heart, which increases your risk for heart attack or stroke.[4]

NERVE DAMAGE

Over time, with elevated blood sugar levels and chronic inflammation, your nerves can become damaged. This condition, called neuropathy, can lead to a variety of symptoms. The most common neuropathy associated with diabetes is peripheral neuropathy, which causes tingling or numbness in your feet, legs, hands, and arms. For some people, this "tingling" eventually turns into excruciating pain. This type of nerve damage affects up to 50 percent of those with type-2 diabetes.[5]

Peripheral neuropathy often leads to ulcers and poor wound healing on the feet or toes, which can lead to amputation if untreated. Another complication of this type of sensory or motor nerve damage is the loss of coordination and balance. Often, those with neuropathy in their lower extremities are prone to falls, which can be dangerous.

In addition to diabetic peripheral neuropathy, there are other types of nerve damage that can affect people with high blood sugar. Autonomic neuropathy is the second most common type of nerve issue with diabetes, affecting the nerves that control the digestive system, heart, and sex organs. This type of neuropathy can cause gastroparesis, which leads to slow digestion, making blood sugar regulation more difficult.[6]

People with diabetes also have a higher risk for focal neuropathies, such as carpal tunnel syndrome and Bell's palsy. Carpal tunnel syndrome may impact up to 25 percent of people with diabetes.

KIDNEY DISEASE

About 25 percent of people with diabetes will develop chronic kidney disease. When your blood sugar and insulin levels are always high, it damages the blood vessel clusters in your kidneys, leading to thickening and scarring of the nephrons, which affects the way they function to filter waste. The longer this progresses, the more damage the kidneys sustain. Eventually, the kidneys can stop working, leading to end-stage renal disease.

There are other risk factors for kidney disease, including smoking, family history, being overweight or obese, and poor lifestyle choices, but over 40 percent of kidney failure cases are due to diabetes.[7]

VISION LOSS

Another scary consequence of diabetes is a loss of vision. The most common type of eye problem caused by diabetes is diabetic retinopathy, which results from damage to the eyes' small blood vessels. This disruption can start as mild vision impairment, such as blurred vision and difficulty seeing at night, but can lead to total vision loss if not controlled.

Again, the damage to the blood vessels is caused by high blood sugar, increased blood pressure, and chronic inflammation associated with diabetes. Most people who have diabetes for more than thirty years will develop some degree of retinopathy if they don't control their blood sugar effectively.

Retinopathy isn't the only eye problem associated with diabetes. People with diabetes and high blood sugar have twice the risk of developing glaucoma, a condition of increased pressure in the eye leading to damage to the optic nerve. There is also a higher incidence of macular edema, a swelling in the part of the eye that helps us focus. Lastly, people with diabetes are more likely to develop cataracts, a clouding of the lenses in the eyes caused by a buildup of deposits from high blood sugar and inflammation.[8]

MORE EFFECTS OF DIABETES

Other complications of diabetes include hearing loss, Alzheimer's disease and other forms of dementia, skin conditions, depression, and sexual dysfunction.[9]

When diabetes develops, it begins a cascade of adverse metabolic effects, leading to chronic inflammation, cardiovascular disease, microvascular damage in the eyes and feet, damage to autonomic nerves controlling digestion and sexual function, and damage to the brain, causing Alzheimer's disease and other forms of dementia.

Everyone deserves normal blood sugar, but normal blood sugar is not enough. If we lower blood sugar with medication, like reducing fever with an antipyretic medication, we've done nothing to fix the actual problem—and therefore have done nothing to mitigate the potential effects.

JIM'S TRAGIC STORY

I still remember the massive smile on Jim's face. He was one of my first patients in a new office that I had opened on the Main

Line suburbs of Philadelphia after leaving the endocrinology practice. Jim was a sixty-two-year-old man with an incredible spirit. He was a simple man and was willing to do whatever was required to get better. When he came into my clinic, Jim was dealing with severe peripheral neuropathy, and his blood sugar was out of control (his HbA1c was over 10 percent).

When I looked at Jim's feet, they were dry and rough and looked like he didn't give them much attention. I did a neurological exam and found a significant degree of numbness. They also hurt at night, and Jim had been prescribed gabapentin to help with the pain.

After listening to Jim's story, I gave him some recommendations, including significant dietary changes and starting to walk regularly.

Jim was a great patient. He did everything that I asked and more, and he saw great results within just a few weeks.

At his next office visit, he was smiling. His blood sugar was in the low 100s for the first time in years, and his feet no longer hurt. Jim was on top of the world.

The next time Jim was due for an appointment was about a month later. He didn't make it. After seeing my other patients, I called him at home. What he told me broke my heart.

He had started exercising at the gym and hired a personal trainer. A few days later, he noticed a blister on his foot. Within a week, it had turned into a red, swollen mess. A few days after that, his foot needed to be amputated.

Like my experience with Kathy at the endocrinology practice,

I'll never forget that moment. I learned a few things that day, not the least of which is how important it is to take care of your feet, even if things seem right and blood sugar is getting better. The feet are always at a much higher risk for problems with diabetes.

But the biggest lesson I learned from Jim is that diabetes is a ruthless disease. It can destroy your life, steal your vision, or take your foot in an instant. To fight it, we have to be just as vigilant—just as ruthless.

Diabetes is not just high blood sugar, and solving the diabetes puzzle involves much more than just taking blood-sugar-lowering drugs. We have to address the root causes of diabetes and high blood sugar—including chronic inflammation, environmental toxins, dietary and lifestyle factors, sleep and stress, physical activity, and energy toxicity. And it is essential to address the foundational cause of type-2 diabetes, insulin resistance, which I'll discuss more in the next chapter.

CHAPTER 2

THE INSULIN PROBLEM

Insulin is a powerful hormone—a growth stimulator designed to protect the body from running out of fuel. In people whose bodies don't make insulin (such as type-1 diabetics), it becomes impossible to store energy. Everything they eat is used immediately by the body or rapidly excreted through the urine, bowels, breath, and sweat.

Furthermore, without insulin, there is no brake on the constant metabolism of energy substrates. Again, those who don't make enough insulin rapidly waste away, losing their body fat and muscle mass under the unopposed stimulation of glucagon, cortisol, and adrenaline. Insulin protects us.

Under normal circumstances, during times of energy abundance (when lots of food is available), the pancreas releases insulin, which causes the body to save everything. Like during the oil crises of the 1970s when people filled up with extra gasoline so they wouldn't run out, insulin causes the body to save excess energy to protect it from starvation during times of famine. Any glucose not used immediately for energy gets stored as glycogen or transported and packed into fat cells. Amino acids get used for protein synthesis, and the fat cells become locked so they can't release free fatty acids into the bloodstream.

Unfortunately, as we saw in the last chapter, too much of a good thing turns into type-2 diabetes, pre-diabetes, and metabolic syndrome. When insulin levels are too high for too long, we become energy toxic and go into storage overload.

Insulin was first isolated by Drs. Banting, Best, and MacLeod at the University of Toronto in 1921 and used two years later in the first successful treatment of a patient with type-1 diabetes. This "discovery" was a bit controversial because other scientists had discussed insulin years earlier, but the findings were not fully understood. For example, 19th-century physiologists recognized that the pancreas played a crucial role in processing energy in the body. Still, they couldn't figure out the direct role the pancreas played in diabetes until two physiologists removed the pancreas from a dog in 1890.[10]

Once the pancreas was removed, the two scientists observed severe diabetes development in just three weeks. Subsequent studies and experiments over the years supported the conclusion that the pancreas was critically involved in the development of diabetes. Many years later, scientists realized what was inside the pancreas: small clusters of specialized cells termed the islets of Langerhans, where insulin is made.

Named by Dr. Sharpey-Schafer, a London physician who studied the areas of the pancreas that produce the hormone, the term insulin is derived from the Latin "insula," or island, referring to the "islands" of beta cells in the pancreas.[11]

The discovery, isolation, and ultimate production of insulin have been lifesaving to the millions of people with type-1 diabetes who cannot produce insulin. In 1977, medical physicist Rosalyn Sussman Yallow won the Nobel Prize in Physiology for creating a radioimmunoassay test for insulin. Unfortunately, the test, which should have been a game-changer, is seldom used for those with diabetes and blood sugar problems. Despite its widespread availability and low cost, the insulin test has never been adopted into mainstream guidelines and recommendations. The practice of medicine is often slow to change, but hopefully, this test will soon be incorporated into the standard of care for a diabetes evaluation.

THE ROLE OF INSULIN

Many scientists believe that insulin may have originated more than one billion years ago. Apart from humans and other animal species, insulin-like proteins are also known to exist in the Protista (an organism that is not plant, animal, or fungi) and Fungi kingdoms.

As a peptide hormone produced inside your pancreas, which sits just behind the stomach, insulin is considered the main anabolic (promoting metabolic activity) hormone in your body. By promoting the absorption of glucose from your bloodstream into your liver, fat cells, and skeletal muscle cells, it regulates the metabolism of the carbohydrates, fats, and protein that you eat.

Each time you eat—particularly carbohydrate foods, but to a lesser extent, any food—the beta cells in your pancreas are alerted. In response, they secrete insulin to help move sugar and amino acids from your blood into your liver and muscles for use or storage. These cells are very sensitive to blood sugar levels. If glucose levels in the bloodstream are high, they secrete insulin. If blood glucose levels are low, they inhibit the release of insulin.

The body is highly efficient at burning fuel in the form of fatty acids and glucose, either directly by the cells or in the millions of energy factories in the body, called mitochondria. Thanks to insulin, it's also very good at storing energy for later use. A kind of metabolic switch controls this process so that the body is either burning fuel or saving fuel, though not at the same time.

You see, metabolically, you exist in one of two states at any given time: the fed state or the fasted state.

When we eat (fed state), those beta cells in our pancreas recognize that carbohydrates and amino acids have hit the bloodstream, and the production and release of insulin start to increase. The more carbs we eat, the more insulin is released.

But what happens to insulin when we are not eating? Between meals (after about four to five hours) and each night when we're asleep, we shift into a fasted state. That's where things begin to change.

Even when you are not eating, the body requires energy to beat the heart, activate the brain, produce new muscle cells, and release chemicals for optimal body function. So where does your body get the energy to do all that work?

Right next door to the beta cells in the pancreas are alpha cells. These cells take their cue from the beta cells, secreting glucagon when blood glucose is low and decreasing glucagon release when blood glucose is high.

When you haven't eaten for a while, your blood sugar starts to drop, insulin stays low, and the alpha cells in your pancreas are alerted to secrete glucagon to release stored energy from the liver and fat cells.

So when it comes to whether fat gets stored in your body or burned for fuel, insulin is the star of the show. You are either prioritizing fat burning or fat storage, not both at the same time.

This fact is one of the reasons that people have such a hard time losing weight.

When you eat three, four, or five meals per day, and each of those meals has an ample supply of carbohydrates (even if those carbohydrates are from whole foods like fruits, whole grains, and beans), your pancreas will secrete insulin. Remember, insulin will signal your body to store energy in the form of glycogen in the liver and muscles, or in the form of fat in the adipose cells.

Depending on how much energy you've consumed and how much energy you need at that moment, insulin will drive as much glucose as possible into the liver, muscles, and other cells. If there's still some left over, it will activate other hormones that convert glucose into fat to pack the fat cells. That's if everything is working correctly.

Sometimes, it doesn't.

INSULIN RESISTANCE AND HIGH INSULIN LEVELS

Insulin is essential for human life. It is our primary anabolic hormone, causing the body to utilize energy and store excess fuel. Over time, however, this finely tuned system can break down, leading to communication problems within the body.

In the last chapter, I described insulin as a key that opens the doors in the cells, allowing glucose to flow in to be metabolized into energy. In reality, this mechanism is much more complicated. When insulin binds to its receptor on the outside of a cell, it sets off a chain reaction called post-receptor signaling, which ultimately opens a channel called GLUT-4 in muscles, fat, and heart tissue and facilitates the transportation of glucose into the cell.[12]

There are several potential breakdowns in this communication cycle that can lead to insulin resistance.

For example, specific inflammatory cytokines have been shown to interfere with the signaling pathways in the cells that are triggered by insulin. Certain environmental toxins, known as diabetogens or endocrine disruptors, can also antagonize or block the binding of insulin to its receptor, as though they are jamming the lock.[13]

We also know that when glycogen levels get full and the adipocytes, or fat cells, have reached their capacity, the body purposely downregulates insulin sensitivity as an adaptive mechanism.[14] This type of insulin resistance has been referred to as an "overflow phenomenon" due to the energy toxicity that we also discussed in the last chapter.[15]

Unfortunately, the body responds to insulin resistance by making more insulin. This response is called adaptive hyperinsulinemia and leads to high circulating levels of insulin, not only after eating but also between meals and fasting.[16] This phenomenon leads to a constant lock on the fat cells, entirely preventing the body from effectively breaking down stored fat for energy. Additionally, chronic hyperinsulinemia can have harmful effects on all insulin-sensitive tissues—including fat cells, muscles, kidneys, pancreas, liver, and brain.

Nephrologist Dr. Jason Fung has said, "I can make any one of my patients fat by giving them insulin."

There are plenty of studies that have now confirmed this fact. One such study, published in the *American Journal of Clinical Nutrition*, showed that the strongest predictors of weight-loss resistance and weight regain in those who lost weight were insulin resistance, hyperinsulinemia, and inflammation.[17]

Indeed, we know that giving insulin to a patient who is already hyperinsulinemic and insulin resistant will cause significant weight gain. It quickly forces all the extra glucose in their blood into their fat cells. When the fat cells fill, they start storing fat in and around organs like the liver and pancreas, leading to fatty liver disease, metabolic syndrome, and type-2 diabetes.

WHAT CAUSES INSULIN RESISTANCE?

Genetics; age, ethnicity; body weight; fat accumulation in the liver, pancreas, and muscles; lack of physical activity; and specific dietary factors can all contribute to the development of insulin resistance. Let's look at some of the most potent contributors.

CHRONIC INFLAMMATION

Various studies have shown that a chronic inflammatory response, triggering a host of inflammatory cytokines, can cause insulin resistance. These cytokines, like TNF-α, Interleukin-1β, Interleukin-6, and others, interfere with the insulin signaling pathways in the cells, leading to insulin resistance.[18]

Inflammation of the brain and gut can also cause leptin (a

hormone that regulates appetite and metabolism) resistance, leading to insulin resistance.[19]

This chronic inflammation can start in the gut, or it can be a response to trauma, a poor diet, overtraining, or chronic stress.

CONSTANT STRESS AND CORTISOL

When we're stressed, our bodies produce hormones in response. One of these hormones is cortisol. Cortisol plays several essential roles in the body, but its primary function is to raise blood sugar by activating new glucose production and the breakdown of glycogen in the liver. This process gives our body a sudden burst of energy to deal with immediate stress in our environment.

Unfortunately, this stress response in modern society is continuously hyperactivated for many people, leading to chronically high levels of cortisol in our bloodstream, which, in turn, creates high blood sugar. This elevated blood sugar leads to greater insulin demands from the pancreas, which causes hyperinsulinemia and insulin resistance.

Cortisol has also been shown to directly cause insulin resistance of the muscle and liver cells. Its main job is the liberation of energy substrates, so it acts to prevent the liver and muscles from using all the glucose and fat it's activating.

TOXINS

The air we breathe, the water and food we consume, and self-care products like cosmetics and bath products all contain toxins. Each year, our exposure to these toxins grows. Once inside our body, these endocrine-disrupting chemicals cause inflammation and interfere with our glucose and fat metabolism, eventually inducing insulin resistance.

Several studies have described specific toxins, like arsenic, BPA, phthalates, dioxins, and PCBs.[20] Once they get into the body, they can circulate in the bloodstream, causing problems for years. For example, BPA, which has been used in the production of polycarbonate plastics, can block insulin receptors, leading to insulin resistance, elevated blood sugar, and obesity. Some of these chemicals have been phased out in the Western world but persist in the air and ground soil.

ENERGY TOXICITY AND FAT ACCUMULATION

One of the most significant contributors to insulin resistance is the excess stimulation of insulin by overconsumption of energy. When the body wants to store the extra food energy, there is only a limited capacity for glucose (about 80–100 grams in the liver and 300–400 grams in the muscles). Once those are full, which can happen quickly, the body will convert extra glucose to fatty acids and store them in the fat cells under the influence of insulin.

Fat cells, or adipocytes, can expand greatly—up to twenty times their original size. However, at some point, if we continue to overconsume energy, our fat cells will reach their storage limits. Genetic factors largely determine this capacity, which describes a concept called personal fat threshold.[21] When the body reaches its storage capacity for glycogen and fat and exceeds the personal fat threshold, it downregulates insulin sensitivity as a protective mechanism.

We also become desensitized to insulin, similar to how we can become desensitized to chemicals like caffeine, alcohol, and nicotine. When insulin levels are chronically elevated due to a diet high in processed and refined grains and sugars that stimulate massive insulin release, the cells start to turn down their insulin response, decreasing sensitivity and leading to insulin resistance.

Lastly, fat accumulation in and around the organs, such as the liver and pancreas, plus elevated levels of free fatty acids in the bloodstream, have all been linked to insulin resistance. Like toxins, free fatty acids and other compounds such as sphingolipid ceramides, cause insulin resistance by interfering with insulin signaling pathways in the cells.[22]

Ceramides are an important component of cell membranes, but they can be overproduced and accumulate in the cells due to excessive blood fat levels. This process happens when the body is not correctly metabolizing fat after the overconsumption of energy.

HOW TO STOP AND REVERSE INSULIN RESISTANCE

Insulin resistance is the proverbial elephant in the room. Not many doctors want to talk about it because they don't quite understand the mechanisms behind the condition, and not many patients even know the condition exists or that they might have it. So the giant elephant remains in the room, invisible, thrashing about and causing increasing chaos and destruction.

Yet no matter how much we avoid the topic, insulin resistance is a major problem in our culture. It is the root cause of many of the chronic health problems we see today, including obesity, type-2 diabetes, heart disease, high blood pressure, PCOS, fatty liver disease, and Alzheimer's disease and other forms of dementia. It's also been linked to certain cancers like breast and endometrial cancer.

For women, it's also interesting that many of the symptoms attributed to menopause are caused by insulin resistance. Insulin has a cascading effect on all of the other hormones, including estrogen, progesterone, and testosterone. When insulin can't do its job effectively, it is almost impossible to reduce or eliminate the symptoms associated with menopause, including hot flashes and night sweats. It becomes virtually impossible to lose weight.

To reduce or reverse insulin resistance, it is vital to address the various causes discussed earlier in this chapter. By focusing on fixing the root causes of insulin resistance, you can reduce your risk of insulin-related health problems, including metabolic syndrome and type-2 diabetes. Let's take a look at some ways to address these factors.

FAT LOSS (ESPECIALLY ABDOMINAL FAT)

One of the leading causes of insulin resistance is a buildup of fat around the organs, such as the liver and pancreas, and in the blood. The American Academy of Family Physicians has noted a strong correlation between abdominal fat and the degree of insulin resistance, regardless of how much you weigh overall.[23]

A study at Garvan Institute of Medical Research, St. Vincent's Hospital, in Sydney, Australia, found that abdominal fat was a reliable marker for insulin resistance and is most likely the determining factor of insulin resistance in women. The study also reported that a simple measurement—waist-to-hip ratio— was predictive of hyperinsulinemia and insulin resistance.

Some experts argue that there is no way to target belly fat, but research disputes this assertion. Several published research papers have demonstrated that low-carbohydrate diets that minimize insulin secretion produce a proportionally higher level of fat loss from the visceral area (belly) than other diets.[24]

Exercise can also make a big difference. One study at Duke University Medical Center found that non-exercisers experienced roughly a 9 percent gain in visceral fat after six months, while study participants who exercised the equivalent of jogging ten miles per week lost visceral fat as well as subcutaneous fat (fat right under your skin). Strength training for an hour a couple of times a week has shown to be a surefire way to lose stubborn belly fat.[25]

REDUCE INFLAMMATION

Inflammation is another root cause of insulin resistance. In fact, chronic inflammation is the root cause of most of the diseases we're dealing with today, including cardiometabolic disorders, obesity and weight gain, type-2 diabetes, and Alzheimer's disease.

Much of the chronic inflammation that plagues our health begins in the gut. It's been reported that 70 percent of the entire immune system is in the gut, and 80 percent of immune plasma cells reside in the gut.[26] When the gut barrier is damaged or too porous, it sets off an immune reaction that spreads throughout the body.

Avoiding processed and refined foods like sugars, grains, vegetable oils, processed meats, and common food sensitivities like dairy products will reduce the inflammatory response in the gut.

Additionally, studies have consistently shown that a diet rich in anti-inflammatory foods such as fatty fish, which contain beneficial omega-3s, can help reduce levels of inflammation.[27] Other anti-inflammatory foods include berries, cherries, broccoli, avocados, green tea, and spices like turmeric.[28]

REDUCE STRESS AND MANAGE CORTISOL LEVELS

As mentioned earlier in the chapter, the adrenal hormone cortisol that is released on a circadian rhythm and during times of stress has been shown to cause insulin resistance, particularly in the liver and muscles.[29]

Reducing stress is easier said than done. However, there are many strategies that can lower cortisol and help you feel more mentally alert, energized, and healthier when practiced regularly.

Some examples of healthy ways to reduce stress and increase peace include meditation, journaling, prayer, healing bath, meditative walks, mindfulness training, tai chi, and heart rate variability training. Finding the approach that works for you is critical.

ENERGY-RESTRICTED LOW-CARBOHYDRATE DIETS

It's hard to believe that some physicians, dietitians, and diabetes educators think a low-carb diet is dreadful for people with diabetes and insulin resistance or dangerous in some way. That's like saying avoiding gluten is too extreme for those with celiac disease. It makes absolutely no sense.

The fact that carbohydrate-rich foods have the most significant impact on blood sugar levels is well established. The more carbs you eat, the more insulin your body produces and releases into the bloodstream. The more insulin your body releases, the more weight you gain and the more likely you are to develop insulin resistance and type-2 diabetes.

Many studies have shown that a low-carb diet can improve insulin resistance, lower blood insulin levels, increase fat loss, and reverse type-2 diabetes.[30] One of these studies, published in the *Annals of Internal Medicine*, revealed a 75 percent reduction in insulin levels in ten obese patients with type-2 diabetes who followed a low-carbohydrate diet. The authors noted a spontaneous decrease in energy consumption by the participants in the study. In other words, they naturally ate less following the low carb diet approach.[31] So it's clear that if you want to reverse insulin resistance, it's good to reduce the intake of sugar and carbohydrates while also reducing energy intake to improve fat burning.

STRATEGIC FASTING

Scientists have been increasingly studying the effects of fasting on metabolic health, and the results are impressive. A report published in *Nutrition Reviews* looked at time-restricted eating, a type of intermittent fasting, and reported that it improved metabolic health by reducing lipids, lowering blood sugar and fasting insulin, increasing insulin sensitivity, and reducing inflammatory cytokines.[32]

One of the most exciting strategies for lowering insulin levels and reducing insulin resistance is strategic fasting. This type of fasting refers to using specific techniques, like the one described in this book, that reduce circulating insulin levels, increase insulin sensitivity, activate fat loss, and improve blood sugar levels.

I'll describe much more about this later in this book, including some background on the ProFAST diet and substantial research showing the benefits of fasting for diabetes, fat loss, and insulin resistance.

OPTIMIZE ESSENTIAL NUTRIENTS

Our food is not just composed of protein and energy from carbohydrates and fat. It also contains fiber, water, and lots of micronutrients. These nutrients—such as vitamins, minerals, flavonoids, antioxidants, and other phytonutrients—have essential roles to play within the body.

One of the most important of these micronutrients is the mineral magnesium. Magnesium is essential for over 300 biochemical reactions in the body, including nerve and muscle function, immune function, bone health, heart rate, blood sugar metabolism, and mitochondrial function. Additionally, studies have shown that optimal magnesium levels are necessary to prevent insulin resistance.[33]

Coenzyme Q10 is another critical nutrient that helps boost mitochondrial health and acts as a powerful antioxidant, thereby supporting metabolism. Alpha-lipoic acid is an antioxidant that improves the cells' response to insulin and can stabilize blood sugar levels.

Chromium is an essential mineral that helps improve glucose tolerance and insulin response, stabilizes blood sugar, and may improve serum lipid profiles. Several studies have documented the benefits of chromium, especially combined with the B vitamin biotin, to improve blood sugar and insulin levels.[34]

HOW ROBIN FUELED THE FIRE

One of my clients, Robin, had been struggling with her weight and diabetes for many years. When she came into my office, she weighed about 280 pounds and was round and inflated. Her face was puffy. Her ankles were swollen, and her stomach protruded from her body like a balloon.

Exasperated, she told me that it hadn't always been this way. She explained that about eight months prior, she was 160 pounds after losing some weight. Robin had been working with another doctor to clean up her diet and had started exercising. She had been doing much better and felt great.

Then, she lost her sister and became overwhelmed and depressed. Just thirty days after burying her sister and best friend, she gained twenty pounds, and her blood sugar climbed to over 300 mg/dl. Her doctor, out of desperation, told her that she needed to start insulin right away.

Unfortunately, her doctor did not understand the problem—that she had become extremely insulin resistant under tremendous stress. When injecting insulin did little to lower her blood sugar, she was instructed to keep increasing the dose. Six weeks later, she was taking well over 100 units per day of long-acting insulin and another sixty units of rapid-acting insulin. Her weight increased dramatically almost overnight.

By the time she walked into my clinic, she had gained over 100 pounds, and her blood sugar was still over 200 mg/dl on most days. We needed to do something dramatic to get quick results.

I shared the ProFAST diet with Robin, and she enthusiastically agreed to start right away. She went to see her physician, told him that she would be stopping insulin, and asked him to help her monitor her bloodwork and medications. He reluctantly agreed.

After ProFAST, Robin experienced a dramatic change. She was no longer puffy and swollen. Her stomach was no longer protruding from her body, and her skin had a healthy glow. She smiled, feeling free from a life with high blood sugar, diabetes complications, and daily insulin injections.

Eight weeks after starting the ProFAST diet, Robin had lost almost sixty pounds, and her blood sugar had dropped below 100 mg/dl for the first time in ten years. After a short break, she decided to do two more rounds of ProFAST, losing another forty-five pounds and eliminating three additional medications on top of the insulin that she'd discontinued.

Insulin resistance is a complex health condition with a lot of moving parts. The more you understand how insulin works in the body and how to optimize its function, the better you can burn stored fat and avoid the metabolic disaster that excess insulin creates.

CHAPTER 3

ENERGY DENSITY VERSUS NUTRIENT DENSITY

Vegan advocate Dr. Joel Fuhrman is the author of a book called *The End of Diabetes*. One of the key concepts he discussed in the book was nutrient-density, or the number of micronutrients per calorie.[35]

He created something called the ANDI, or the Aggregate Nutrient Density Index. While this seemed like a powerful concept that could be very useful in designing an optimal diet for those trying to lose weight or address type-2 diabetes, something didn't seem right. For example, grains like oats and corn were ranked much higher in nutrient density than meats and eggs, which are packed with nutrition. How could this be?

Well, it turns out that there was an inherent bias that tilted the ANDI toward plant-based foods and away from animal products. For example, the ANDI focuses heavily on carotenoids, phytosterols, glucosinolates, angiogenesis inhibitors, and organosulfides, which are mainly found in plant foods. It ignores amino acids, cholesterol, carnitine, choline, and omega-3 fatty acids, which are higher in animal products.

Marty Kendall, an engineer whose wife has type-1 diabetes, was able to rework the data and create a more comprehensive scoring system for nutrient density, which he published on his website.[36]

When looking at his analysis more closely, many vegetable foods like leafy greens and herbs still top the nutrient-density chart, but animal foods like shellfish and whitefish follow them. Whole grains, it turns out, are some of the most nutrient-poor foods available, and it gets much worse when they are processed and refined.[37]

There are a total of forty essential nutrients that the human body needs plus water. These include nine essential amino acids, two essential fatty acids, thirteen essential vitamins, and sixteen essential minerals. In addition to these, there are various beneficial compounds, such as polyphenols, flavonoids, carotenoids, antioxidants, sulforaphanes, and other helpful nutrients in plant and animal foods.

When we evaluate the amount of these nutrients compared with the energy provided in the form of fat and carbohydrates from various foods, it forms a scale of nutrient versus energy density. The more nutrient dense and less energy dense a particular food is, generally, the better that food will be for optimizing weight loss and metabolic health.

WHY DO WE EAT?

In essence, we eat to provide our bodies with the energy to fuel our bodily functions and the raw materials that we need to build and repair tissues—including muscles, organs, enzymes, hormones, neurotransmitters, and other biochemicals. Energy comes mostly from the carbohydrates and fat in our food, and the raw materials come from protein and micronutrients. So if we analyze the major components of our food, we can break them down into two classes: energy and nutrients.

Both are essential, and many scientists believe that we continue to eat until we get enough protein and nutrients from our food.[38] If you were to eat only protein, however, your brain and body chemistry would force you to seek energy-rich foods. Otherwise, you would succumb to a condition known as "rabbit starvation," which was first described in explorers who tried to survive on ultra-lean rabbit meat alone.[39]

It's the balance of these two food components, energy and nutrients, that ultimately determines whether we stay lean and healthy or accumulate fat and become obese and metabolically sick.

Of course, there are many other reasons people eat besides the energy and nutrients we can extract from our food. In an article published in the *Journal of Clinical Endocrinology and Metabolism*, the authors described "Hedonic Hunger" as the "consumption of food just for pleasure and not to maintain energy homeostasis."[40] A term coined by Dr. Michael Lowe at Drexel University, hedonic hunger has been blamed on the availability of hyper-palatable, energy-rich foods that essentially hijack our taste buds and brain to overconsume.

Eating can also become habitual. Various studies have indicated that the human brain can become conditioned to eat highly pleasurable foods and to crave foods at certain times based on habit.[41] If you snack at night, you'll feel the "need" to continue to snack at night because you've established a habit.

We also eat for social reasons, including a feeling of connection with others, family bonds, cultural norms, peer pressure, and social anxiety.

Lastly, many people eat for emotional reasons. This pattern may happen because they are bored, stressed, depressed, or sad. We often look to food for comfort instead of addressing the root emotional issues leading to this type of hunger. Certain foods, such as refined sugar, gluten, casein, and flavorings, can have powerful effects on the addiction centers of the brain, triggering the same responses that opioid drugs like morphine do.[42]

This fixation can lead to compulsive overeating, binge eating, and other types of emotional eating in many people. A study published in the journal *Nutrients* found that almost 20 percent of overweight women were diagnosed with food addiction using the Yale Food Addiction Scale.[43]

According to the SAMHSA, a division of the U.S. Department of Health and Human Services, there are several triggers for addictive behavior such as emotional eating. These include "negative feelings," such as fear, anger, and shame; "normal feelings" like boredom, embarrassment, and frustration; and "positive feelings" such as celebration and confidence. It's best to identify the specific triggers that seem to affect you the most and create an action plan and avoidance strategy.[44]

Overcoming food addiction, compulsive eating, social eating disorders, habitual eating, and hedonic eating is essential so that you can train your body to eat for energy and nutrients, focusing on the ideal dietary breakdown for optimal health.

WHAT ARE HUMANS SUPPOSED TO EAT?

Talk about a loaded question. When you ask anyone what the ideal human diet is, including trained dietitians, you'll likely get a wide array of answers. There are few topics on which there is less consensus than this one.

However, some generally accepted facts about human nutrition can help guide our understanding of what we should be eating.

Plants are "autotrophs," concentrating energy from the sun, air, and soil into stored energy. They pull together chains of carbon, hydrogen, oxygen, nitrogen, and other essential nutrients to form their structure and functional components.

When animals eat plants, they concentrate the elements in these plants to form energy and functional nutrients. This process is called bioaccumulation and biomagnification and is the reason animal foods are often more nutrient dense than plants.

Herbivores, such as cows and deer, only eat plants. These animals have large flat teeth and digestive tracts designed to break down large amounts of plant material and often ferment it into short-chain fatty acids.

Carnivores are on the opposite end of the food chain and eat other animals almost exclusively. These include wild cats and sharks. These animals typically have sharp teeth and simple digestive systems.

Lastly, there are omnivores, which eat a variety of food sources, including plants and animals. Humans are omnivores, as are bears and chickens. Omnivores have both sharp and flat teeth and have more complex digestive tracts.

As omnivores, humans can thrive on both plant and animal food sources. We can concentrate the energy and nutrients that we need directly from plants or use the substrates already extracted by other animals. Interestingly, plants seem to store most of their energy as carbohydrates, while animals save their extra energy, typically as fat.

ENERGY-TO-NUTRIENT BALANCE

As we've discussed, humans (and other animals) eat to extract energy and nutrients from their food, and they eat until they obtain enough energy, protein, and micronutrients to build and maintain their structure and function.[45]

During our evolutionary history, there were periods when food was not readily available, marked by severe energy restriction. Hence, we evolved to be able to store energy effectively to use during times of low-energy states.

The two primary energy sources for human metabolism are fat (broken down into fatty acids and stored as triglycerides) and carbohydrates (broken down into sugar and stored as glycogen). While the human body can store some sugar in the form of glycogen in the liver and muscles, storage capacity is limited. On the other hand, fat can be stored almost without limitation, and the average person has a one-hundredfold increased capacity for fat storage over sugar. Once our glycogen stores are full or near capacity, the body shifts to storing all extra energy as fat.

As mentioned earlier, conditions like type-2 diabetes, metabolic syndrome, and obesity are forms of energy toxicity.[46] Chronic overconsumption of high-energy foods overfills our fat cells. We become adapted to store fat in the organs, viscera, and muscles, leading to increased insulin resistance, dyslipidemia, and metabolic dysfunction.

This high-energy, nutrient-deficient diet, termed the Standard American Diet (SAD), has now been adopted by most of the world to varying degrees. While many hunter-gatherer populations consume 30–35 percent protein, the average older American is only getting sixty-six grams of protein per day, or about 13 percent of their caloric intake.[47] This level of protein consumption is woefully deficient and, combined with the diet's energy-rich, nutrient-poor aspects, is likely contributing to the escalating rates of obesity and diabetes around the world.

While low in protein, today's highly processed, hyper-palatable foods tend to be rich in both carbohydrates and fat. This distribution is not matched, however, in whole natural foods. In fact, it's difficult to find any whole foods that are high in both fat and carbohydrates, with the exception of mammalian milk and some nuts.

This phenomenon was described in the book *Don't Eat for Winter* by Cian Foley.[48] There, Cian discusses how certain animals—such as squirrels during autumn—will purposefully fatten themselves for winter by eating a diet rich in carbs and fats. When the squirrel gorges on acorns, the macronutrient ratio almost precisely matches that of typical American cuisine, such as donuts, milk chocolate, potato chips, and ice cream.

The problem here is that eating carbohydrate-rich foods forces us to burn sugar preferentially because we have limited storage capacity for it. This propensity then displaces fat oxidation—meaning, we are not burning fat. So when we eat a large amount of fat combined with high carbohydrates in the same meal, all that energy is immediately stored as body fat. Additionally, since we can't store the extra fuel from the high-carbohydrate meal as sugar, the body converts it to fat to store in our adipose tissue.

This trapped energy from overconsumption of low-nutrient foods is the leading cause of obesity, type-2 diabetes, and metabolic syndrome in America and worldwide.[49] Excess energy gets captured in the body, leading to toxicity, inflammation, insulin resistance, hyperlipidemia, and elevated blood sugar.

Losing weight, burning fat, restoring insulin sensitivity, and reversing chronic metabolic disease can only occur when we eliminate the energy toxicity and restore balance to our metabolic system.

Here is a list of foods with the highest energy density compared with those with the highest nutrient density. Focusing on foods with a higher nutrient density will help balance the amount of energy we consume with the proper amount of protein, fiber, and micronutrients, which is essential to creating optimal metabolic health.

ENERGY-DENSE FOODS

- Refined oils
- Refined sugar
- Cheese and full-fat dairy
- Fried foods
- Ice cream
- Soda and juice
- Granola and breakfast cereals
- Milk chocolate
- Dried fruit
- Whole and refined grains

NUTRIENT-DENSE FOODS

- Leafy green vegetables
- Herbs
- Asparagus
- Broccoli and cauliflower
- Seafood (oysters, crab, lobster)
- Fish (haddock, halibut, salmon)
- Seaweed
- Liver
- Whole eggs
- Pork chop and chicken breast

THE FAT SQUIRRELS

Earlier, I mentioned the anti-autumnal diet described by Cian Foley in *Don't Eat For Winter*. The nutrient and energy consumption pattern that squirrels and bears follow during the fall to prepare for winter, unfortunately, mirrors our standard American diet. This begs the question: what happens if winter never comes?

In 2016, we were able to see.

November and December of 2015 were unseasonably warm in many areas of the world that would otherwise see cold temperatures. The abundant food supply for the squirrels never ran out, and in January and February of 2016, people started noticing that there were a *lot* of fat squirrels.

Fortunately for the squirrels, according to scientists, they eventually stopped overeating and assumed their average size and weight by the following year.

As humans, we live in a never-ending autumn, with an abundance of high-energy food available at all times and no impending winter to use it up. All we need to do is walk over to the refrigerator or pantry, stop by the fast-food restaurant on the way home from work, or grab a soda and snack from the vending machine. We have become a society of fat squirrels, and we need to do something about it before it's too late.

CHAPTER 4

PRIORITIZING PROTEIN

At the end of 2017, I received a message from a woman named Francine. She responded to a video interview that I had released with a plant-based cardiologist named Dr. Joel Kahn. Joel is a friend of mine, and even though we disagree about specific dietary strategies, we had an open, honest, and lively discussion about the role of nutrition in diabetes prevention and reversal.

After reading a story about the unethical treatment of animals, Francine had been a vegan for just over a year. She wrote that she had worked with a plant-based dietitian to construct her vegan diet and included plenty of plant protein, whole grains, vegetables, and supplements for missing nutrients, such as vitamin B12.

In the beginning, she told me, things went well. She felt more alert, had more energy, and noticed improvements in her digestion. However, after about a year, things started to take a turn for the worse. First, she noticed that her energy had waned. Even though she was going to bed early and sleeping through the night, she was tired all day and needed to nap to survive. Even with the naps, she was starting to feel exhausted around the clock.

She also noticed that her blood sugar became very irregular—high at times and low at others. Her gut, which had improved at the beginning, wasn't doing well either. She was experiencing gas, bloating, and stomach pains often.

The dietitian she was working with put her on iron supplements, encouraged her to take high-dose vitamin C, gave her some adrenal supplements, and told her to drink more fluids. None of it worked.

Finally, she went to a different nutritionally focused doctor who encouraged her to add back some animal protein. Francine said that she was scared and felt somewhat ashamed at first but reluctantly tried it. After about a week of eating fish, eggs, and grass-fed beef, she started to notice a difference. Her energy improved. The bloating in her stomach disappeared, and she wrote that she "felt alive again."

Months later, Francine said she accepted that her body just needed some "real protein" and that a restrictive vegan diet was not for her.

For every Francine, I'm sure there are others who feel like a plant-based diet has changed their lives for the better. It can be done, and I've helped some of my patients improve their metabolic health and even reverse type-2 diabetes while following a plant-based diet. But it's a more difficult path. One study found that 84 percent of the people who tried following a vegan or vegetarian diet went back to eating meat.[50]

There are many reasons for this, from social stigma and conflict to disappointment and difficulty, but the most significant reason is negative health consequences. As I described in the previous chapter, human beings are omnivores. We have evolved to eat plants and animals to extract the energy and nutrients we need to thrive. By cutting out animal products, the vegan eliminates an entire category of natural, whole foods, which in some ways are nutritionally superior and more nutrient dense than most plant foods.

Thriving on a vegan diet is like trying to play golf with only a putter and a few irons. You can do it, but it's going to be a lot more challenging.

To optimize metabolic health long term, we need to prioritize protein. And that is most effectively accomplished through an omnivorous diet.

WHY DO WE NEED PROTEIN?

In the macronutrient world, protein doesn't get all that much attention, especially compared to fat and carbohydrates. We hear things like, "Saturated fat causes diabetes and heart disease, while carbohydrates are essential," or "Carbs make you fat and lead to diabetes, while fat is healthy."

With the exception of bodybuilders who watch their protein consumption faithfully, most of these discussions center on carbohydrates and fat. Most people don't give much thought as to why eating optimal protein is imperative or which are the right sources to promote their overall well-being and metabolic health.

Yet proteins are the "building blocks of life," responsible for constructing your entire body, including your muscles, cells, hormones, neurotransmitters, and detoxification substrates.

Without adequate protein, the body would quickly deteriorate and die.

Proteins are organic molecules made up of twenty different amino acids, with nine of them considered essential amino acids. Because the body cannot manufacture them, we need to get them through our diet. These include histidine, isoleucine, leucine, lysine, methionine, phenylalanine, threonine, tryptophan, and valine.

Then there are the nonessential amino acids that the body can usually make for itself. I say usually because there are some health conditions (including stress) that can affect the body's ability to make what it needs. The nonessential amino acids are alanine, asparagine, aspartic acid, and glutamic acid. Some amino acids are considered conditionally essential because they become essential under periods of extreme trauma and stress. These include arginine, cysteine, glutamine, tyrosine, glycine, ornithine, proline, and serine.

Without adequate protein intake, your body can't and won't function properly, let alone optimally.

Protein helps to create new cells to replace old, worn-out cells. It aids in the growth and repair of your body's muscle tissue and organs. It helps produce essential chemicals in the body, such as enzymes, neurotransmitters, hormones, and antibodies. And the amino acids from protein can be used, in a limited capacity, to produce energy.

In the previous chapter, I discussed the energy-to-nutrient balance and shared that conditions like obesity, type-2 diabetes, and metabolic syndrome are typically states of energy toxicity.

The energy gets trapped in the fat cells, organs, and muscles from years of over-consumption of high-energy foods, leading to increased insulin resistance and metabolic disease.[51]

When we look at our meal composition and the energy-to-nutrient balance within it, the most abundant and significant nutrients for metabolic health are the amino acids from protein. Additionally, protein content in food typically increases as nutrient density increases. In most cases, the higher the protein percentage of the food, the more nutrient dense it tends to be.[52]

In his book, *The P:E Diet* (which stands for protein-to-energy ratio), Dr. Ted Naiman lays out a clear case for increasing protein and reducing energy in the diet to optimize metabolic health.

He also discusses the "protein leverage hypothesis," coined by Drs. Raubenheimer and Simpson from the University of Sydney. These doctors noticed that from 1961 to 2005, the average protein percentage in the American diet dropped 14 percent to 12.5 percent, which led to an increase in energy consumption by almost 15 percent.[53] While there are certainly other factors, like gastric distention and hormonal signals, humans will generally continue to eat until they get the nutrients they need from their diet, regardless of the energy content of the food. This fact often leads to overconsumption of energy due to the protein dilution of the modern diet, leading to obesity, type-2 diabetes, and other metabolic problems.[54]

According to Dr. Naiman, getting enough protein is one of the keys to reducing energy consumption, burning more fat, eliminating insulin resistance, and optimizing metabolic health. The protein-to-energy ratio is defined as the grams of protein in a food compared to the grams of fat and net carbohydrates. An ideal protein-to-energy ratio for health and weight maintenance is 0.5–1.0 grams of protein per gram of energy.[55] To increase fat burning and encourage fat loss, the protein-to-energy ratio should be over 1.2.

Examples of high P:E ratio foods include fish, seafood, chicken, leafy green vegetables, plain (low-fat) Greek yogurt, lean ground beef, cruciferous vegetables, steak, and eggs.

PROTEIN AND WEIGHT LOSS

Protein is incredibly important when it comes to losing and maintaining a healthy weight. Consuming protein increases our levels of a hormone called glucagon, which activates fat burning.

As glucagon increases and insulin decreases, free fatty acids are liberated from fat stores to provide energy for the muscles and organs. This is the process our bodies were designed to do—store fat when food energy is in abundance and burn fat when food energy is scarce. Reducing energy consumption in the form of fat and carbohydrates and increasing the consumption of protein helps your body burn stored fat.

Protein also helps the body lose fat through a mechanism called the thermic effect of food, or TEF. This term refers to the increase in metabolic rate, which is the rate at which your body burns energy when you eat.

In other words, the very act of digestion can increase how much energy you burn, based on the kind of food you eat or, to be more specific, based on the energy content and macronutrient composition. Not all foods have the same TEF, and protein uses the most energy.

The TEF of protein, or the energy dissipated by digestion, is about 20–25 percent of the total potential energy in that food. Carbohydrates have a TEF of 5–10 percent, and fats are significantly lower at 0–3 percent. This difference means you burn far more energy digesting protein than carbohydrates or fat.[56]

Protein-rich foods are also known to be more satiating than most foods high in refined carbohydrates or fat. When we eat more protein, we feel fuller longer, helping us to eat less overall. This idea is based on research on the "satiety index" of foods developed by Australian researcher Dr. Susanna Holt from the University of Sydney. In her 1995 study, she measured how full people felt after consuming a fixed calorie load from a variety of foods.[57]

A study published in *Obesity* showed that eating more protein (25 percent of dietary caloric intake) resulted in less desire to eat at night, less snacking, reduced obsessive thoughts about food, and an increased feeling of fullness.[58]

Another study, done at the University of Washington, found that people who ate a 30 percent protein diet ended up consuming almost 450 fewer calories each day as opposed to those who ate a 15 percent protein diet.[59]

Increased protein consumption has also been shown to reduce weight regain after an energy-restricted diet. This phenomenon is something we'll discuss more in the maintenance chapter later in this book.

Various studies have established the connection between higher protein consumption and improved lean body mass.[60] Additionally, higher protein consumption protects muscle from breakdown during fat loss on an energy-restricted diet. This protection and preservation of lean body mass is one of the most significant benefits of adequate protein consumption and an optimal protein-to-energy ratio.

When protein levels dip too low, the body will break down skeletal muscle and other lean body mass, like the heart, to use for energy production. This process can lead to a significant loss of muscle tissue and cardiac complications in people trying to lose weight on low-protein, energy-restricted diets.[61]

The more muscle mass we have as humans, the higher our capacity for glycogen storage and fat and glucose disposal through mitochondrial oxidation. The most effective way to increase metabolic health and flexibility is to improve our oxidative capacity by building more lean body mass. In other words, protein consumption drives muscle synthesis.

HOW MUCH PROTEIN SHOULD YOU EAT?

The DRI (Dietary Reference Intake) for protein is 0.8 grams per kilogram of body weight or 0.36 grams per pound.

This intake amounts to only fifty-six grams of protein per day for the average man and a measly forty-six grams per day for the average woman. Though this meager amount may be enough to prevent deficiency leading to protein malnourishment, studies show that it's far from sufficient to ensure optimal health and body composition.[62]

Dr. Osama Hamdy, in the Department of Endocrinology at

Harvard University, has suggested that 1.5–2.0 grams of protein per kilogram of ideal body weight, or 20–30 percent of caloric intake, may be better for those trying to lose weight or control type-2 diabetes and blood sugar. In one paper, he stated, "There is increasing evidence that a modest increase in dietary protein intake, above the current recommendation, is a valid option toward better diabetes control, weight reduction, and improvement in blood pressure, lipid profile, and markers of inflammation." He also noted that increasing protein led to substantial reductions in hemoglobin A1c.[63]

Another recommendation, from Drs. Schoenfeld and Aragon, in the *Journal of the International Society of Sports Nutrition*, stated that based on the current evidence, optimal protein consumption for muscle health should be 1.6–2.2 grams per kilogram of body weight.[64]

As energy toxicity expert Dr. Naiman states, you quite literally are what you eat. If you want to have more fat, eat more energy. If you want to have more muscle and be leaner, eat more protein.

I'll discuss macronutrient distribution and calculation later in this book when I explain the details of the ProFAST diet.

WHAT ABOUT THE RISKS OF HIGH PROTEIN?

For people with normal kidney function, there is minimal risk of consuming too much protein. There is a far higher risk of a *deficiency* in protein, especially in older adults, by not getting enough to protect lean body mass and metabolic health.

The Institute of Medicine recommends a wide range of 10 to 35 percent of daily energy intake to come from protein.[65] For the average male, this would equate to an upper limit of about 218 grams of protein per day, and for the average female, about 174 grams of protein. Other studies have shown that adults can tolerate up to 3.5 grams of protein per kilogram of body weight without adverse side effects. In an 80 kg (176 lb) person, this would equate to about 280 grams of protein per day.[66] Greenlandic Inuit, who get almost 45 percent of their calories from protein, eat almost precisely 280 grams of protein per day and have done so for many decades without liver or kidney problems.[67]

If you were to go above these limits, there are potential risks related to the overconsumption of protein. Like with any nutrient, including water and many vitamins, overeating can cause problems. Excessive protein intake can lead to the overproduction of ammonia, urea, homocysteine, and nitric oxide.[68] Overconsumption of arginine, an amino acid, can lead to gastrointestinal distress due to a high nitric oxide synthesis rate. High protein consumption may increase GFR by 5 percent in the kidneys to process the nitrogen load, although there has been no evidence of harm to the kidneys or dysfunction reported in those with normal kidney function.[69]

A few minor consequences are reported with higher-protein diets, including dehydration, bad breath, and constipation.[70] These may be partly due to the production of ketones, leading to the expiration of acetone. These can be remedied by drinking more fluid and consuming vegetables high in fiber and water content.

WHAT ABOUT PEOPLE WHO HAVE KIDNEY DISEASE OR GOUT?

There is evidence that in people with stage one, two, or three chronic kidney disease (CKD), it may be beneficial to limit protein consumption to 15 percent of total caloric intake.[71] That's about 93 grams of protein for a man and 75 grams for a woman. Interestingly, those numbers still exceed the average protein consumption of most older Americans. For stage four CKD, protein may be limited to 10 percent (62 grams for men, 50 grams for women), and in stage five, everything changes due to the need for kidney dialysis.

If you are prone to gout or have high uric acid levels, you may want to consider eating low-purine foods. Purines are healthy and necessary organic compounds that form the building blocks of our DNA. But during detoxification, they are broken down into uric acid and are responsible for about 15 percent of the uric acid in the body. When excessive uric acid builds up in the blood, it can lead to kidney stones, gout, and other problems.[72]

The foods highest in purines include beef, bacon, wild game meats, organ meats, oats, beans, nutritional yeast, and some seafood, including tuna, sardines, anchovies, herring, mussels, codfish, scallops, trout, and haddock. Alcohol, like beer and whiskey, and fructose (from fruit and added sources) are also known to raise uric acid levels.

PROTEIN MYTHS

The fear of overconsumption isn't the only myth circulating about protein. This nutrient is often completely ignored or, worse, gets an entirely undeserved lousy reputation by the nutrition community. Here are a few more common myths that people have heard about protein.

MYTH #1: YOU ONLY NEED HIGH PROTEIN IF YOU ARE A BODY BUILDER

This misconception is not even close to accurate. Protein builds and protects muscle and lean body mass. It constructs your entire body, including bones, joints, tendons, ligaments, hair, skin, antibodies, hormones, enzymes, and the LDL and HDL carriers for cholesterol. Plus, protein helps support a healthy immune system and helps regulate blood glucose.

Increasing protein and decreasing energy (from carbohydrates and fat) is a surefire way to burn more body fat and improve metabolic health, no matter who you are.

MYTH #2: OVEREATING PROTEIN CAUSES KIDNEY DISEASE

I've discussed this in detail above. In summary, excess protein consumption only has the potential to be a problem if your kidneys are already progressing through disease or are failing.

If you have healthy kidney function, protein is completely safe within the limits that I recommended earlier. Your kidneys are entirely able to expel the extra nitrogen that comes from eating lots of meat, eggs, and fish without adverse effects.

MYTH #3: EVERYONE SHOULD TAKE A PROTEIN SUPPLEMENT

For most people, getting enough protein through diet is not only possible but preferred. While I'm all for a healthy and delicious protein smoothie, this type of protein gets absorbed and digested very quickly, which may actually raise insulin levels slightly.

If you are a vegan or vegetarian or have a hard time getting enough protein from your food, supplementing it with a good-quality protein powder is fine. For most people, though, it's just not necessary.

If you decide to use a protein supplement, make sure it's a high-quality, professional product, free of artificial ingredients, added sugars, and contaminants.

MYTH #4: ALL PROTEIN IS THE SAME

The protein in plants is not the same as the protein in meat, eggs, fish, and other animal products. Animal sources of protein are the most bioavailable for our bodies and are "complete proteins" because they contain all nine essential amino acids. Plant-derived proteins, with a few exceptions, do not include all essential amino acids, so you have to get more creative with your food selection to optimize your nutrition.[73]

I recommend choosing the best-quality sources of animal products (or plant proteins) that you can find and afford. Commercially raised beef and poultry contain more contaminants, hormones, and inflammatory fats than their grass-fed and pastured counterparts. Likewise, farm-raised fish are often dyed in color and have higher levels of pollutants (such as mercury) and inflammatory omega-6 fats than wild-caught fish.

SKINNY ISN'T EVERYTHING

I came across a book several years ago called *Muscle Up* by author PD Mangan. In the book, he made a case for resistance training to prevent cancer, heart disease, and other chronic diseases, such as type-2 diabetes.[74] I enjoyed the book and found it helpful but found the author's story even more compelling.

Dennis (PD) Mangan has formal training in pharmacology, biochemistry, and microbiology. His health journey was similar to many others, as he followed the standard health advice from his doctor to eat a low-fat diet, do aerobic exercise for fitness, and keep an eye on his cholesterol levels. And it worked—on a surface level. The problem was that despite being skinny on the outside, he wasn't feeling very well and was getting sick.

After getting nowhere with his doctors and ultimately getting worse, he decided to turn to his knowledge in health, biochemistry, and research to fix himself.

He started eating more protein and cut down on the processed carbs that are so common in the diet today. He began lifting weights and doing various forms of resistance training. He established a routine to build more lean body mass, increase his testosterone, and reverse the aging process.

I recently had the pleasure of interviewing PD Mangan for my *Mastering Blood Sugar* podcast. At sixty-plus years old, he is now healthy, lean, and muscular, and he reports having more energy, increased libido, and better metabolic health than at any point in his life.

Working with thousands of patients and clients over the years, I've found that there is no more significant impact on blood sugar, insulin resistance, and metabolic health than replacing some of the energy in your diet, especially carbohydrates, with more protein.

Protein makes us feel more satiated, protects and helps build muscle and lean body mass, increases the body's metabolic rate and energy expenditure, and fuels many processes in the body, including detoxification and neurotransmitter production, enzyme activity, and protein synthesis.

When in doubt, for optimal blood sugar and metabolic health, cut the carbs, cut the fat, and eat more protein.

CHAPTER 5

THE POWER OF FASTING

Fasting is, perhaps, the ultimate energy-restricted dietary strategy. The intentional abstention from food has been used for thousands of years to improve health, eliminate disease, increase energy, extend life, and enhance cognition.[75]

Fasting is included in almost every spiritual discipline to overcome physical desire and get closer to spirit. It's been used safely and effectively, in various ways, as a therapeutic strategy by physicians and philosophers such as Hippocrates, Plato (400 BC), and Plutarch (100 AD) and continues through the current day.[76]

Additionally, fasting has been integrated into our evolutionary biology as a regular and expected event throughout human history. According to Yale food historian Dr. Paul Freedman, PhD, "Up until about 12,000 years ago, all humans got their food by hunting, gathering, or fishing. As foragers, they would fast until they found, caught, or killed their food. There was no breakfast upon waking or leftovers for lunch. They ate opportunistically, consuming anything they could get their hands on."[77]

The body is hard-wired to survive periods without food and to increase healing, repair, and recovery. Aligning to that natural pattern may lead to better health and longevity.

The Scottish *Postgraduate Medical Journal* relays an interesting story of one man's experience with fasting. Published in 1976, the case report describes the experience of a man named Angus Barbieri, who lost 276 pounds and reduced his blood sugar levels substantially in a little over one year while fasting. When Angus started his supervised fast, he weighed 456 pounds.[78]

During the 382 days of fasting, he was allowed to have only water, coffee, tea, seltzer, and some vitamins and minerals. When he broke his fast over a full year later, he weighed just 180 pounds. At the five-year follow-up, the researchers reported that he had maintained his weight loss and health improvements.

In the published article, the researchers described several other fasting case reports lasting between 210 and 256 days, with one report of periodic fasting lasting 350 days. They stated that the rate of weight loss for Angus (0.72 pounds per day) was similar to that in the other case reports (0.41–0.67 pounds per day).

The most exciting thing about Angus's story is that he reported feeling in good spirits throughout the yearlong fast. Indeed, he ultimately determined the length of his treatment—choosing to fast until he reached his goal of 180 pounds.

So how is it possible for some people to skip food for an entire year, while others get "hangry" if they miss one meal?

Certainly, Angus initially had ample fat storage to last him while he wasn't eating, but as he got closer to his goal, that may not have been the case. Yet his hunger completely dissipated as he fasted, and he even reported forgetting how food tasted. When he broke his fast with a hard-boiled egg, he told the reporter, "I thoroughly enjoyed my egg, and I feel very full."

Let's look at what happens during a fast that allowed this man to live over a year without food, and that may be a clue to health for many of us.

THE FASTING AND FED STATES

If you could look inside your body and see what's going on beneath the surface, you would be amazed. Countless actions are in motion at all times, without us even being aware of them. These activities change throughout the day, depending on what we're doing. For example, the physiology of the body shifts substantially between when we are eating and not eating. These patterns are known as the "metabolic states of the body," and include the absorptive, or "fed" state, the post-absorptive, or "fasted" state, and the starvation or "long-term fasted" state.

According to Smith and Morton, British medical professors and authors of *The Digestive System*, the most crucial factor driving the body's metabolic state is the secretion of the hormone insulin.[79] When we eat, the pancreas releases insulin, which dictates the reactions we know as the absorptive or fed state. When we stop eating, insulin levels fall, and we enter the post-absorptive or fasted state.

Understanding how the body transitions from eating to not eating is vital to realizing the benefits of fasting and how the body adapts to periods of energy restriction. During the fed state, we are breaking down food, using it for energy and storing the excess. Alternatively, during the fasted and long-term fasted states, we are breaking down that stored energy to fuel the brain and body.

Regardless of where the fuel comes from (through the diet or from stored energy), we need some kind of fuel, including glucose and fatty acids, to run the body. The key to understanding how the body can go long periods without eating is knowing how we break down stored energy and how the body and brain shift their energy requirements.

The fed state typically lasts about four hours, and a lot is happening during that time. The digestive system—including enzymes in the mouth and small intestines, hydrochloric acid in the stomach, and millions of microorganisms in the gut—go to work on our food, breaking it down into sugars, amino acids, fatty acids, fiber, and micronutrients. As those macronutrients enter the bloodstream, the pancreas releases insulin to signal incoming energy. The liver and muscles also go to work, absorbing the sugar to burn for energy or store as glycogen and amino acids to use for protein synthesis. Anything left over gets converted to fat and sent to the fat cells (adipose tissue) to be stored.

The high insulin levels associated with the fed state encourage the adipocytes to absorb fatty acids and package them with glycerol as triglycerides in a process known as de novo lipogenesis.

In the fasted or post-absorptive state, which starts about four hours after eating and lasts up to twenty-four hours, the body shifts to stored energy as its primary fuel source. This process is, once again, driven by the hormone insulin.

As glucose levels drop, insulin levels continue to fall as well, and the pancreas releases the hormone glucagon, which mobilizes the body to break down stored energy. Most of the glucose needed for the brain, muscles, and cells comes from stored sugar in the liver, called glycogen.

Among its other roles, insulin is a potent inhibitor of lipolysis (the breakdown of fat). So as insulin levels continue to fall, the adipocytes dump fatty acids into the bloodstream to be used as fuel by the body, and we burn more stored fat. During this state, not much else changes, as the body still has ample fuel from stored glycogen and free fatty acids to meet its energy needs.

As the fast continues, beyond eighteen to twenty-four hours (depending on your glycogen stores in the liver and activity level), the body starts to run out of glycogen and needs to start producing glucose in the liver—a process called gluconeogenesis. The primary substrate or source for gluconeogenesis is amino acids from protein, which comes from a process called proteolysis, or the breakdown of protein. The protein used for the production of this energy in the liver comes mostly from non-muscle sources such as the skin and the gut lining to preserve lean muscle mass.[80]

Meanwhile, certain parts of the body start to change their fuel preferences as the fast continues. For example, the muscles stop burning sugar and start burning fat almost exclusively. Further, the heart and brain begin to turn away from sugar and use ketones for energy.

According to Dr. George Cahill, considered the father of fasting research, during the first few days of a prolonged fast, the body will break down about seventy-five grams of protein from muscle to drive glucose production in the liver. The remainder of the glucose requirements come from the breakdown of fat (the glycerol backbone of triglycerides). Fortunately, this level of muscle breakdown doesn't last long. Because the body wants to preserve its muscle mass for movement and strength, it switches to a different fuel as soon as it can: ketones.

Ketones are produced in the liver when insulin levels are low and glucagon levels are high for a prolonged period. As mentioned previously, due to low insulin levels, the fat cells start dumping free fatty acids into the bloodstream. Some of these fatty acids are broken down for energy in organs like the muscles, while others begin to build up in the liver.

With a low level of glucose and glycogen available and an abundance of free fatty acids, the liver starts to produce ketone bodies, called acetoacetate and beta-hydroxybutyrate. These ketones, which I'll discuss more in the next chapter, provide an alternative fuel source for organs like the heart, muscles, and brain. After four days of fasting, approximately 75 percent of the brain's energy is derived from the oxidation of ketones.[81]

As the body continues to fast, growth hormone levels increase, ketones continue to rise, gluconeogenesis slows, and the body starts to burn mostly fat for fuel, conserving lean muscle. Studies from Cahill and others indicate that during prolonged fasting (after about five days), protein breakdown is reduced to just fifteen to twenty grams per day, and up to 90 percent of the body's energy needs are met by fat oxidation.[82]

BENEFITS OF FASTING

While it's fascinating and encouraging to see how the body adapts to prolonged fasting, most people do not want or need to engage in this type of total food abstention. Numerous studies on alternate-day fasting and other intermittent fasting strategies have shown tremendous benefits of shorter fasts—including weight loss, blood sugar control, appetite and craving reductions, lipid improvements, hormone balancing, and cancer prevention.[83]

IMPROVED INSULIN SENSITIVITY

Fasting is one of the most profound ways to improve insulin sensitivity and reduce insulin resistance. We've already seen how insulin resistance and elevated insulin levels lead to weight gain, chronic inflammation, cardiovascular disease, metabolic syndrome, type-2 diabetes, and Alzheimer's disease. And there is no better way to lower insulin levels and improve insulin sensitivity than fasting.

A study in the *Journal of Applied Physiology* found that alternate-day fasting led to a dramatic increase in insulin sensitivity.[84] They found improvements in not only insulin levels but also adiponectin and leptin, which modulate inflammation and appetite. They also reported that fasting in other studies led to a sevenfold increase in insulin sensitivity and may reduce diabetes incidence.[85]

INCREASED METABOLIC RATE

One of the most common misconceptions reported about fasting is that it slows the metabolic rate. While that may be true for prolonged fasting, studies on shorter fasts and intermittent fasting show the opposite. As insulin levels drop during the first seventy-two hours of fasting, other hormones—such as cortisol, adrenaline, and growth hormone—increase to promote the breakdown of fat. These hormones stimulate the central nervous system, often causing a burst of energy and increasing metabolic rate by 3–14 percent.[86]

A study done using alternate-day fasting, published in the *American Journal of Clinical Nutrition*, showed that the participants lost 4 percent of their fat mass with no reduction in metabolic rate.[87]

On the other hand, early studies by Benedict and others found that prolonged fasting may decrease the metabolic rate by 20–30 percent.[88] However, much of this reduction of resting energy expenditure may be related to the weight loss that often accompanies prolonged fasting. Studies indicate that if you lose weight, your metabolic rate will slow down proportionally, no matter how you lose weight. Lighter bodies burn less energy.[89]

WEIGHT LOSS

One of the most exciting things about fasting is that it helps reduce the dangerous fat around the midsection, which can drive inflammation and metabolic problems. Not only does fasting help reduce weight because you are eating fewer calories each day, but it also enhances hormone function, which, in return, facilitates weight loss.

This improvement happens because insulin levels are reduced, as discussed earlier, while growth hormone and noradrenaline levels rise. This burst of stimulation increases the breakdown of body fat for energy.

In other words, fasting helps you lose weight in two ways: it reduces the amount of energy that you're consuming and boosts your metabolic rate at the same time.

IMPROVEMENTS IN METABOLIC HEALTH MARKERS

Multiple studies have shown positive benefits of fasting in lowering blood sugar levels and HbA1c percentage, improving cholesterol and triglyceride levels, improving blood pressure, and reducing oxidative stress.[90]

Fasting increases growth hormone and adiponectin, which protect lean muscle mass, improve insulin sensitivity, and decrease chronic inflammation. Fasting also reduces other inflammatory markers—such as CRP, IL-6, and TNF-alpha—which leads to improved metabolic health and insulin signaling.[91]

Oxidative stress is what ages the human body and causes many chronic diseases. Like rust on a car's bumper or the browning of an apple, oxidative stress is what happens when unstable molecules (free radicals) react with other vital molecules in your body, like protein and DNA, and damage them. Studies show that fasting can enhance the body's resistance to oxidative stress, which can protect that delicate genetic material in your DNA and slow the aging process.[92]

BRAIN HEALTH

Besides reducing oxidative stress and inflammation, as well as blood sugar levels and insulin resistance, research has suggested that fasting is good for brain health. Several studies have found that fasting seems to improve memory and cognitive function and may protect the brain from dementia. Studies indicate that intermittent fasting increases brain glutathione levels, reduces oxidative stress in the brain, and increases BDNF, which may protect the brain from Alzheimer's disease.[93]

PREVENTION OF CERTAIN TYPES OF CANCER

While more human studies are needed, animal studies suggest fasting has several beneficial effects on metabolism that may reduce the risk of cancer.[94] There is also some evidence that suggests fasting can potentially reduce the side effects of chemotherapy in human patients.[95]

INCREASED AUTOPHAGY

Autophagy literally means self-eating. It's a process where the body breaks down old or damaged cell structures and recycles the proteins and other components. It turns something old into something new. This process was first discovered in 1966 and later described by Dr. Yoshinori Ohsumi, who was awarded the Nobel Prize in Physiology.[96]

The cleaning out of "junk proteins" through autophagy has been associated with longevity and reduction in metabolic disease risks, such as cancer and Alzheimer's disease. It has also been proposed to protect pancreatic beta cells from destruction in diabetes.[97]

As insulin falls and glucagon levels increase, autophagy is upregulated, leading to protein breakdown and recycling. Eating less in general (energy restriction) has long been known to increase longevity and improve metabolic health.

Many researchers have described autophagy as the mechanism behind this phenomenon.[98] Various studies have found that energy restriction upregulates AMPK, which induces autophagy.[99]

THE THREE TYPES OF FASTING

Many people cringe when they think of the idea of fasting. The thought of fasting conjures all sorts of imaginary fears. Many people ask, "How could I go an entire day without eating?" and are concerned that they'll starve, have no energy, or shut down their bodies. None of this happens, of course, when you fast.

The truth is that you've been fasting your whole life. Indeed, you fast every day. If you stop eating at eight o'clock in the evening before going to sleep and eat breakfast at eight o'clock the next morning, you fasted for twelve hours. That's half the day!

Fasting is often more of a mental challenge than a physical one. It's one reason that fasting has been used by monks and religions throughout the years to get closer to God. By overcoming the physical desire to eat and letting go of the mental chatter that you experience around food throughout the day, something powerful happens. Many people report peace of mind and strength of spirit that comes with fasting, which is hard to find otherwise.

There are several types of fasting, based on the length of fast, kind of fast, and fasting schedule. These strategies can be used separately or together to increase the benefits of energy restriction and fasting.

TIME-RESTRICTED EATING

For a novice faster, the easiest way to begin is simply extending your overnight fast a few hours. Perhaps that means cutting out the snacks at night and finishing your last meal by eight o'clock. It could also mean delaying breakfast until ten o'clock in the morning or later. By extending the overnight fast, you are practicing something called "time-restricted eating." TRE has been shown to offer tremendous benefits for metabolic health, blood sugar, and weight reduction.[100]

By shrinking the window of time that you're eating, you will naturally eat less, and many people find that it helps them control their appetite and break the snacking habit.

Another variation on TRE is called early time-restricted feeding, or eTRF. With this approach, you eat first thing in the morning, typically within one hour of waking, and stop eating in the early afternoon. The "eating window" might be from eight o'clock in the morning to two o'clock in the afternoon, with a "fasting window" that continues the rest of the day through the next morning. One study on eTRF showed superior blood sugar-lowering benefits, reductions in HbA1c and lipids, and improvements in other metabolic health markers.[101]

These patterns of TRE are often referred to as 12:12, 16:8, or 18:6 based on the number of hours you are fasting and eating in a given twenty-four-hour day. Time-restricted eating can be followed every day or scheduled throughout the week, incorporated into an intermittent fasting strategy.

INTERMITTENT FASTING

As the term implies, intermittent fasting means that you fast for a certain period, followed by eating and fasting again. Typically, intermittent fasting refers to a period of greater than twenty-four hours. There are various IF strategies that can be used to improve metabolic health, reduce food intake, and encourage weight loss and better blood sugar.

One method, created by author Michael Mosley, is called the 5:2 diet. Using this approach, you would fast for two days each week and eat regularly the other five. These days can be back-to-back days but are typically staggered, with a few days of eating between them. This strategy can be done as a full water-only fast or as an energy-restricted day with 500–800 calories, as Dr. Mosley typically recommends. He has written several books about this approach, including *The Fast Diet*, and has reported excellent results with his method.[102]

Another approach to intermittent fasting, which has been studied extensively, is called alternate-day fasting. With ADF, you will typically fast for a full twenty-four-hour period and then eat regularly during the next twenty-four hours. This schedule can be repeated every other day or done two to three times per week. In some cases, the fasting period is extended to thirty-six to forty hours for a deeper fast with even more significant benefit. Studies on alternate-day fasting show multiple benefits, including increased fat loss, improved blood sugar and HbA1c levels, reduced cholesterol and triglycerides, less inflammation, and enhanced cognitive function.[103]

This approach is often recommended and used by nephrologist, diabetes specialist, and author Jason Fung, MD. In his books, including *The Obesity Code*, he describes the benefits of fasting to improve insulin sensitivity, burn fat, and reverse type-2 diabetes.[104]

As I discussed earlier in the chapter, the liver will typically exhaust its glycogen stores within eighteen to twenty-four hours, depending on the size and capacity of the liver and activity level. Extending the fast beyond twenty-four hours forces your body to upregulate fat burning as your body shifts to fat as the primary fuel source.

PROLONGED FASTING

Throughout medical history, there are countless case reports of the powerful benefits that come from prolonged fasting. A prolonged fast typically refers to a fast longer than forty hours and can extend for days or weeks. Any extended fast should be medically supervised, as there are many considerations, such as health status, medications, and lab findings. Often, electrolytes need to be replenished, and lab tests, such as uric acid, need to be monitored closely.

Most people will never need or want to do a prolonged water-only fast. However, there are situations where this strategy can be transformational and lifesaving. Certain autoimmune conditions, severe obesity, and other inflammatory conditions have responded well to prolonged fasting.

There are a variety of strategies that employ energy restriction to achieve many of the same benefits conferred by full fasting as an alternative to short- or long-term water-only fasting.

FASTING ALTERNATIVES

One fasting alternative, called the "fasting-mimicking diet," was created by researcher Valter Longo of the University of Southern California. Dr. Longo studied the benefits of fasting, including upregulation of autophagy, and wanted to find a way to replicate these findings without having to fast completely. His research uncovered an eating strategy that did precisely that. Using the fasting-mimicking diet, you eat about 500–700 calories per day for four to five days in a row, once per month.

According to studies on the FMD, this strategy leads to better glucose control, improved fat loss, reductions in lipid levels, and improvements in HbA1c, and it may even revive pancreatic beta cells, reversing diabetes.[105]

Another strategy, which I'll discuss in more detail later in the book, was created by a researcher named Roy Taylor. His approach uses an energy-restricted diet of about 500–700 calories per day for eight weeks to reverse type-2 diabetes. Dr. Taylor has published multiple papers describing the benefits of his approach, including fat reduction in the liver and pancreas, normalization of blood glucose levels, reduction in blood pressure, and the elimination of diabetes medication.[106]

Finally, I'll be discussing a similar strategy in this book, called the protein-sparing modified fast. PSMF uses an energy-restricted diet approach, based on meeting the necessary protein requirements to prevent the breakdown of lean muscle tissue while fasting. This strategy has been studied extensively over the past fifty years for rapid fat loss and reversal of type-2 diabetes and metabolic syndrome.[107] Notably, it's been used by the Cleveland Clinic in their metabolic health department and validated through dozens of clinical research trials.[108]

the ProFAST diet is an adaptation of the protein-sparing modified fast I've used for years with my private clients to achieve tremendous blood sugar and metabolic health results. We've seen hundreds of my patients and clients reduce fat, particularly the fat around the midsection and organs, normalize blood sugar levels, and reverse type-2 diabetes so they no longer require diabetes medications.

We'll be exploring the ProFAST diet and the protein-sparing modified fast in detail later in this book.

THE FINAL KEY

Several years ago, an article appeared in *Reader's Digest*, sharing eight remarkable stories about people who had reversed type-2 diabetes using fasting. In this article, the writer discussed the work of Dr. Jason Fung, whom I mentioned earlier, and some remarkable transformations seen from fasting.[109]

One of the people in the article, a social worker named Jill, was diagnosed with type-2 diabetes at age thirty. After living in denial for many years, she eventually started on insulin. Unfortunately, her weight continued to increase to over 300 pounds. When she stumbled upon the ketogenic diet and Dr. Fung's work and began to practice intermittent fasting, sometimes fasting as long as seventy-two hours, she lost over 100 pounds, normalized her blood sugar, and reversed type-2 diabetes. She said, "I believe fasting was the final key to heal my metabolic illness of diabetes."

John was also featured in the article. He had been over 400 pounds, struggling with type-2 diabetes, metabolic syndrome, high blood pressure, sleep apnea, and acid reflux. His conventional doctor was pushing insulin injections, but John wanted to follow a different path. After starting his fasting regime and adopting a low-carbohydrate diet, he lost 160 pounds, was able to eliminate most of his medications, and got off his CPAP machine. He reported that his blood sugar, HbA1c, and lipids were normal, and he reversed his insulin resistance and type-2 diabetes.

Fasting has been used for millennia as an effective strategy for health restoration. Contemporary studies have shown powerful benefits from complete and modified fasting strategies, including increased fat loss; normalization of blood sugar and HbA1c; reductions in cholesterol, triglycerides, and other atherogenic lipids; enhancement of cognitive function and brain structure; and reductions in chronic inflammation. Fasting also upregulates autophagy, which may prevent cancer and lead to disease reduction and longevity.

This approach should not be a secret. Fasting is a safe and effective way of optimizing blood sugar and insulin levels and, in many cases, reversing type-2 diabetes. There are several options for short- and long- term fasting using complete food abstention or energy-restricted regimes to achieve the remarkable and transformative benefits of fasting while minimizing or eliminating the drawbacks.

That's the essence of this book, *The ProFAST Diet*, and later I'll describe this method of effective fat loss to normalize blood sugar levels and reverse type-2 diabetes. Before we get there, let's explore in more detail the magic of ketones.

CHAPTER 6

THE MAGIC OF KETONES

For most of our medical history, scientists have believed that the human brain depends entirely on glucose for fuel, burning 100–150 grams of glucose daily. This idea was widely accepted as fact until researchers in the 1960s started putting together some ideas around an alternative fuel source.

Starvation studies uncovered that the amount of protein breakdown based on nitrogen excretion diminished over time. They reasoned that in the absence of dietary carbohydrate, there must be something feeding the brain other than the glucose produced through the glucogenic breakdown of protein. This was known as the "starvation paradox."

If the brain were to depend solely on glucose produced using the amino acids derived from the catabolism of muscle protein, it would need a pound of muscle every two days, leading to rapid sarcopenia (loss of muscle) and death.

In 1966, Dr. George Cahill, whom I described in the previous chapter, reasoned that ketones, including acetoacetate (AcAc) and beta-hydroxybutyrate (BHB), might be the alternative fuel source feeding the brain.[110] In a 1967 landmark study, Cahill and his colleagues determined that the brain derives 35–50 percent of its energy requirements from ketones after a few days of fasting and shifts to 60–70 percent after about a week, thus solving the starvation paradox.[111]

The production of ketones by the liver during low energy states, they found, serves to protect the body from lean muscle loss and preserve glucose for red blood cells and parts of the eyes, which can only metabolize glucose for energy.

For many years before Cahill's work, ketones were considered "undesirable byproducts of incomplete fat oxidation."[112] This discovery rebranded ketone bodies from villain to hero.

Ketone bodies had been first identified in the latter part of the 19th century in the urine of diabetic patients who were in a diabetic coma.[113] When an insulin-dependent diabetic (usually type 1) does not have enough insulin in their body, the hormone glucagon signals the rapid, unopposed breakdown of fat (lipolysis), leading to massive ketone production.

Since ketones are mildly acidic, a buildup in the blood to very high levels can lead to a condition called acidosis (diabetic ketoacidosis or DKA). Some of these ketones will be dumped by the kidneys with large amounts of glucose and can be detected in the urine.

For another fifty years after their discovery, ketones were demonized as the potential cause of severe diabetic reactions and death. After the work of Cahill's team, ketones got a new life and some redemption. Another researcher, Dr. Richard Veech, published several studies following Cahill's work, describing the many benefits and therapeutic uses for ketones. He found that during low energy states, not only the brain but the heart relies primarily on ketones for fuel. He described ketosis as a "critical evolutionary development" to protect the human brain during periods of low energy consumption.[114]

Building on this understanding of ketones and the brain, Dr. Russell Wilder of the Mayo Clinic first proposed the ketogenic diet in 1921 for children who have epilepsy. Dr. Wilder's therapeutic diet is very low in carbohydrates and high in fat, with adequate protein and calories to sustain growth.[115] The ketones seem to have both a pharmacological and metabolic effect on the brain, leading to a decrease in seizure activity.[116]

A study done at Johns Hopkins University in 1992 validated this approach, with 67 percent of the patients showing improvements in seizure control. Further, the ketogenic diet was both effective and sustainable, with a high rate of compliance.[117]

HOW KETONES ARE FORMED

Once thought to be dangerous byproducts of a faulty metabolism, we now know that ketones are highly efficient metabolic fuel during low-energy states because of their ability to be quickly burned by a wide variety of tissues with limited oxygen.[118] They are easily transported into cells due to their water-soluble nature and oxidized in the mitochondria, yielding up to ten times as much energy as glucose metabolism.

The formation of ketone bodies, known as ketogenesis, occurs in the mitochondria of liver cells (and to a lesser degree in brain cells) in response to a low-glucose, low-insulin environment and an increase in fat breakdown. When insulin levels are low and glucagon levels rise, fatty acids are oxidized, or broken down, into a compound called acetyl-CoA.

In high school biology class, you probably learned about the Krebs cycle (citric acid cycle) and the electron transport chain. These are the assembly lines in the mitochondria that turn the substance acetyl-CoA from fat and glucose into oxaloacetate, producing energy along the way.

When the Krebs cycle gets backed up due to a depletion of oxaloacetate (which gets used up for gluconeogenesis), the acetyl-CoA molecules accumulate, stimulating ketogenesis. This shortage of oxaloacetate can come from low-energy states, such as fasting and energy-restriction, vigorous exercise, very low-carbohydrate diets, and certain medical situations.[119]

Ketones are then dumped from the liver into the blood as beta-hydroxybutyrate and travel to the muscles, heart, brain, and other tissues to be oxidized for energy.

THE DOSE MAKES THE POISON

Swiss physician Paracelsus noted in the early 1500s, "All things are poison, and nothing is without poison; the dosage alone makes it so a thing is not a poison."[120] In other words, in certain amounts, anything, including water, can be toxic.

In diabetic ketoacidosis (DKA)—a severe, pathological state—the liver produces massive amounts of ketone bodies due to an absolute or relative lack of insulin and high glucagon levels. The effects of cortisol and adrenaline often exacerbate this during high-stress periods. During DKA, blood ketone levels often rise to extreme levels, such as 23.0 mmol/L.[121] This situation leads to dehydration and acidosis, which can be dangerous and sometimes even fatal.

In comparison, normal ketone production from an overnight fast rarely exceeds 0.5 mmol/L. Those following a well-formulated ketogenic diet, as described by Dr. Stephen Phinney, will typically have blood ketone levels of 0.5–2.0 mmol/L.[122] During prolonged water-only fasting, blood ketone levels will naturally increase, as described above, to levels of 4–7 mmol/L to preserve lean muscle mass and spare glucose. This level of blood ketones has been extensively studied and found to be safe and protective for the brain and heart.[123]

THE KETOGENIC DIET FOR FAT LOSS AND DIABETES

For thousands of years, our biological ancestors have had access to limited foods. They didn't eat Doritos, ice cream, frozen dinners, or soy burgers.

What they ate was very simple: meat and plants. Depending on the season, the part of the world, and the availability of food, they ate mostly fish or other animals, starchy tubers, non-starchy vegetables, and some fruit, nuts, and seeds. It was all organic, wild-caught, and local. Their diet was naturally high in protein (in most cultures) and contained healthy fats. More importantly, it did not include processed or refined foods like sugars, grain flours, and seed oils. Hence, they were virtually free of metabolic diseases.

If you look at the average person's diet today, it's the complete opposite. Most people eat food high in refined carbohydrates and fats and are deficient in nutrients, with moderate amounts of protein. Chronic diseases like heart disease, obesity, Alzheimer's, cancer, and diabetes have skyrocketed, and this can be directly linked to humans eating the complete opposite of what our bodies need to function optimally.

Most people have been told repeatedly that carbohydrates are necessary for health. Without carbs, we're told, the brain can't function, and we'll die. From a young age, we are taught that carbohydrates give us the energy we need to get through our day.

The truth, however, is very different. In a letter to the editor of the *American Journal of Clinical Nutrition*, entitled, "Is dietary carbohydrate essential for human nutrition?" Dr. Eric Westman writes, "In exploring the risks and benefits of carbohydrate restriction, I was surprised to find little evidence that exogenous carbohydrate is needed for human function."[124]

That doesn't mean that we don't need glucose, however. As discussed earlier, specific cells like red blood cells and parts of the eye do not have mitochondria and cannot burn fat. Their only fuel source comes from the breakdown of glucose in the cells. The key is that we can produce 100 percent of our glucose requirements in the liver from stored glycogen and gluconeogenesis from amino acids, glycerol, and other substrates. So, technically, we don't need to eat any carbohydrates.

It's also likely that the body thrives when burning fat as its primary fuel source. We have limited storage capacity for glucose as glycogen. An average 154-pound (70-kilogram) male stores about 100 grams of glycogen in the liver at full capacity and about 400 grams in their muscles.[125] The muscle glycogen is reserved mainly for the muscle itself, so we are limited to about 400 kcal worth of energy from stored liver glycogen. That's not much.

Fat, on the other hand, is stored much more efficiently and yields a lot more energy. The average person carries 150 times as much stored energy in their fat cells, and one gram of fat yields over twice as much energy as a gram of glucose.

Lastly, glucose is a "dirty" fuel that generates far more reactive oxygen species (ROS) than fat. Fat is a cleaner-burning fuel and produces far fewer free radicals. Think of burning sugar like trying to heat your home by burning newspaper in a wood-burning stove. You could do it, but you'd need to continually add more paper to the fire, which would produce a lot of soot. However, you could burn hardwood instead and generate much more heat without all the pollution. That's like burning fat in your mitochondria.

What we eat mainly determines what fuel our bodies burn. In the presence of an abundance of carbohydrates, the body will burn the sugar and store the fat.[126] When you eat fewer carbs, you allow your body to switch over to its preferred fuel source—fatty acids. If you have extra fat stored on or in your body, it probably makes sense to get better at burning fat. That's one of the main benefits of the very low-carbohydrate ketogenic diet.

The ketogenic diet has garnered a lot of attention over the past few years. Once an obscure treatment for epilepsy, it's become a popular approach for weight loss and blood sugar control. It's a diet that closely mimics how our ancestors ate, focusing on foods high in fat (healthy fats), moderate amounts of protein, and very low in carbohydrates.

As discussed earlier, restricting carbohydrate consumption lowers insulin levels, leading to increased fat breakdown. After a few hours, your body starts to produce ketones. As you continue this eating strategy, ketone production increases, and your body moves into a state referred to as nutritional ketosis. These ketones supply energy to your muscles, heart, and brain while sparing lean muscle and glucose.[127]

Due to the carbohydrate restriction, ketogenic diets often lead to rapid improvements in blood sugar levels, reduce circulating insulin and decrease insulin resistance, speed fat loss, lower triglycerides and total cholesterol, lower blood pressure, and reduce inflammation.[128]

Studies done by Dr. Sarah Hallberg and her team at Indiana University have shown impressive results with pre-diabetes and type-2 diabetes using a short- and long-term ketogenic diet.[129]

In a one-year trial, participants with type-2 diabetes, on average, lowered HbA1c from 7.6 percent to 6.3 percent, lost over thirty pounds (12 percent of body weight), and reduced medications substantially. Ninety-four percent of patients who were prescribed insulin either reduced or stopped their insulin use. A follow-up two-year study found similar results with a combined 70 percent rate of type-2 diabetes reversal and remission.[130]

Another study, published in the journal *Pediatrics*, evaluated over 300 subjects with type-1 diabetes following a very low-carbohydrate (ketogenic) diet. The average HbA1c of the group was 5.67 percent, and they reported a minuscule rate of adverse events in the patient population.[131]

Other studies on the ketogenic diet have shown a reduced risk of heart disease, cancer, Alzheimer's disease and epilepsy and reversal of polycystic ovarian syndrome (PCOS).[132]

HOW TO ENCOURAGE KETOGENESIS

Ketones are naturally produced as an adaptation to low-energy states and carbohydrate restriction. This period includes states of prolonged fasting and energy restriction. As described earlier, extended fasting can lead to blood ketone levels far above normal physiological ranges. While this can feed the brain and reduce muscle loss, this high level of ketone bodies is not necessary to achieve benefits from ketosis.

Most of the studies referenced in this chapter were done using a ketogenic diet low in carbohydrates and relatively high in fat with moderate protein consumption. This diet increases the production of ketones, providing energy to the muscles, heart, and brain without the necessity for full fasting.

Consuming high amounts of fat is not necessary to induce ketogenesis; it can be achieved with the restriction of carbohydrates and overall energy alone. Moreover, if you already have a significant amount of stored body fat, it may be preferable to burn the fat from your adipose tissue, viscera, organs, and muscles instead of supplementing extra fat in the diet.

Proponents of the ketogenic diet will sometimes note that dietary protein can suppress ketogenesis. This effect is real in some situations but may not have a significant contribution.[133] While the addition of circulating ketones has been shown to produce benefits such as reduced appetite, an additional energy source, and suppression of inflammation, the main goal of an energy-restricted diet is to reduce insulin resistance by increasing visceral and hepatic (liver) fat loss.

ARE EXOGENOUS KETONES HELPFUL?

If ketones in the blood can provide such a beneficial effect on metabolic health, you might be wondering if it's a good idea to supplement them. This topic is a new area of research that has led to mixed results.

First, let me explain what the term exogenous ketones means. In medicine, the term endogenous refers to substances produced within the body, such as endogenous insulin production (made by the pancreas). Exogenous refers to substances that come from outside the body. Exogenous ketones are typically formulations of the ketone beta-hydroxybutyrate that have been stabilized and packaged as a supplement.

Exogenous ketones currently come in two forms, which are ketone salts and ketone esters, or a combination of both. Ketone salts are more commonly available and are a combination of BHB and a mineral ion, such as sodium.

Unfortunately, there is little to no clinical research on these products. One study, published in the journal *Applied Physiology, Nutrition, and Metabolism*, showed that supplementing with BHB ketone salts increased fatty acid oxidation during exercise but impaired exercise performance.[134]

Recently, researchers at Diet Doctor set up an experiment with the help of founder Dr. Andreas Eenfeldt to test various exogenous ketone salt products. The results were discouraging. They found that not only did the ketone products offer little to no benefit; they barely raised blood levels of beta-hydroxybutyrate.[135]

The other formulation of exogenous ketones is called ketone esters, which are made by combining the ketone body with a ketone precursor. Although these findings look more promising, there is still a lack of good scientific evidence showing significant benefits of ketone esters.

One study in the *Journal of Physiology* showed that ingesting ketone esters before an oral glucose tolerance test improved glucose and insulin response without impacting other hormone levels.[136] Another study in *Cell Metabolism* showed that ketone esters led to greater exercise performance and increased fatty acid oxidation in muscles.[137]

There needs to be more research in this area before we know if these relatively new products are beneficial. We know currently that endogenous ketone production in the liver, stimulated by fasting, low-carbohydrate diet, and reduced-energy states, provides tremendous benefits to metabolic health.

The ketones help spare glucose and lean muscle, and the metabolic shift that occurs to yield a ketogenic state leads to increased fat burning, reductions in blood sugar and HbA1c levels, lower inflammation markers, and enhanced cognitive function.[138]

THE EXCITING RESEARCH OF DR. SARAH HALLBERG

I met Sarah Hallberg in a small mountain hotel in Breckenridge, Colorado. After skiing the previous day, I raced down to the conference room, still a bit sore, to catch her lecture at a low-carbohydrate conference that I was attending.

That day, she shared the research that she and her team at Indiana University were doing using a ketogenic diet and regular coaching on outcomes in a group of patients with type-2 diabetes. As she explained her protocol, I became increasingly excited because it was almost exactly what I had been doing with my patients and clients for the past five years.

To Dr. Hallberg's credit, she took the important and valuable step of quantifying and publishing the data from her trials, for which I am incredibly grateful.

In 2017, she and her team published a paper in the *Journal of Medical Internet Research* (JMIR) showing a 1 percent reduction in HbA1c in just ten weeks using a ketogenic diet (with an average BHB level of only 0.6 mmol/L). In addition, patients lost an average of over 7 percent of their body weight, and 56 percent had medications reduced or eliminated in that same time frame.[139]

A year later, Dr. Hallberg published another study in *Diabetes Therapy* that summarized the results of her program after one year. The paper showed more favorable benefits, including a reduction of HbA1c from 7.6 percent to 6.3 percent, weight loss of over thirty pounds on average, and, most impressively, a significant decrease in medication use. Remarkably, 94 percent of patients on insulin at the beginning of the study had their insulin reduced or eliminated during the year.[140]

These results echoed what I had been seeing in my private practice and coaching program for years and validated the exceptional results that our clients achieved. I waited for Dr. Hallberg in the hallway and spoke to her for another hour about the program she was using and the research she was doing. She told me that they weren't done, and her group had a two-year and five-year follow-up plan, plus additional studies on the effects of the ketogenic diet on fatty liver disease and sleep.

In 2019, her team published a two-year follow-up study in the journal *Frontiers in Endocrinology* that showed improvements in HbA1c, fasting glucose, fasting insulin, blood pressure, triglycerides and other lipids, weight and fat mass, and liver enzymes. Additionally, the group's use of diabetes medications declined from 55.7 percent to 26.8 percent, and over 70 percent achieved type-2 diabetes reversal or remission.[141]

Dr. Hallberg's work will leave a long legacy and hopefully open the minds of doctors, clinicians, and researchers to the tremendous benefits of ketones and ketogenic diets for metabolic health. I'm certainly grateful to have met her and for the conversations that we've shared.

Ketone production is a healthy adaptation to fasting and low-energy, low-glucose, and low-insulin states. These specialized molecules are uniquely metabolically efficient and fuel the brain, heart, and muscles with an alternative and potentially superior energy source. There are several ways to induce ketogenesis, including the ketogenic diet, prolonged and intermittent fasting, and energy-restricted eating strategies like the ProFAST diet.

In the next chapter, I'll describe how the ProFAST diet works and how to use this enhanced version of the protein-sparing modified fast to burn fat; normalize insulin and blood sugar levels; reduce hemoglobin A1c, lipids, and inflammation; and reverse type-2 diabetes.

CHAPTER 7

INTRODUCING THE PROFAST DIET

What can a humble Brit who runs an MRI research center in the historic city of New Castle in northeast England tell you about reversing diabetes that your doctor or endocrinologist doesn't already know?

Meet Dr. Roy Taylor.

Professor Taylor is the embodiment of what you might imagine a diabetes researcher to be. He's lean and fit with a passion for cycling. He's clearly intelligent, with a dry wit and an unassuming demeanor. Most of all, he's dedicated to his work, writing, and research.

It just so happens that Dr. Taylor's research is focused mainly on type-2 diabetes. More specifically, it's focused on reversing diabetes.

Professor Taylor tells of how, in 2006, he was reading through a scientific journal and stumbled upon a paper on the reversal of type-2 diabetes following bariatric surgery. He says what was striking about the case study was how quickly the patient's blood sugar returned to normal.

That same year, Dr. Taylor had started a research project at New Castle University, with high-tech MRI scanners, substantial funding, and a brilliant team of scientists.

He had a theory about the causes of insulin resistance and high blood sugar associated with type-2 diabetes, and he set out to disprove it. That's what proper research does: it starts with a theory and then tries to prove it wrong with well-designed clinical trials.

In this case, he hypothesized that insulin resistance, which drives the majority of type-2 diabetes cases, is caused by an accumulation of fat in the liver and pancreas. Moreover, if you can reduce this fat by restricting energy in the diet, you could reverse many type-2 diabetes cases.[142]

This new paper on bariatric surgery reinforced his theory. You see, it turns out that the surgery itself didn't cause the drop in blood sugar, but the sudden reduction in eating did. Over the past fifteen years, Professor Taylor has continued studying the mechanisms involved in this phenomenon, steadily proving his theory that type-2 diabetes is reversible in many cases with strategic dietary changes.

The method Dr. Taylor uses in his research is very similar to the process described in this book. We've seen similar results in the thousands of people who have safely and effectively followed this approach. Let's walk through it together.

WHAT IS THE PROFAST DIET?

How would you feel if you could drop 15 percent of your body weight, reduce your blood pressure, and optimize your glucose and triglyceride levels while eliminating diabetes medications or insulin?

Would it be worth following an energy-restricted diet and putting in some effort for a few weeks?

The ProFAST diet is a six-week program to optimize blood sugar levels, reduce liver and visceral fat, and reverse type-2 or pre-diabetes using a therapeutic eating plan based on the protein-sparing modified fast.

In 1973, scientist and physician George Blackburn, while at MIT, wrote a PhD thesis called, "A New Concept and Its Application for Protein-Sparing Therapies."[143] This paper was the birth of what he later termed the protein-sparing modified fast.

As described in the previous chapter, while there are many fasting benefits, one of the most significant drawbacks is a loss of lean body mass during extended fasts.

While this effect is diminished in obese people, there is still a significant loss of lean body mass during prolonged fasts.

Dr. Blackburn, with the help of colleagues such as Dr. Bruce Bistrian, set out to solve this dilemma by creating and researching a method that would protect lean body mass while reducing fat and improving metabolic health.

In 1985, Drs. Blackburn and Bistrian carried out an extensive study to test their protein-sparing modified fast on 668 overweight people. The results were astonishing. On average, the patients, of which 84 percent were women, lost between forty-five and fifty-nine pounds without a reduction in lean body mass (men lost more than women). Also, they saw a substantial drop in blood pressure, blood sugar, and triglyceride levels.[144]

In another study on patients with type-2 diabetes, Blackburn's group found that the protein-sparing modified fast reduced insulin and blood sugar levels substantially. Remarkably, all participants were taken off insulin injections after just seven days.[145]

The Cleveland Clinic has also been studying the use of the protein-sparing modified fast in people with type-2 diabetes and obesity.[146] They published several papers outlining the benefits, including the following:

- Significant weight loss in overweight individuals, leading to a reduction of central adiposity.
- Significant decreases in fasting blood glucose.
- Decreased use of diabetes medications and insulin.
- Significant reduction of HgA1c (up to 3 percent).
- Decreased fasting insulin and reduction of insulin resistance.
- Decreased triglycerides and increased HDL.
- Lower blood pressure and discontinuation of blood pressure medications.
- Improved kidney function and reduction of kidney markers.

The protein-sparing modified fast is considered one of the most effective diet strategies to reduce stubborn fat and blood sugar. Yet it is seldom used or discussed by mainstream medical physicians.

If there were a pharmaceutical drug that conveyed these benefits, with little to no side effects, how many doctors would prescribe it?

How many patients would line up to take it?

The most exciting part about this program is that it's not complicated. As you'll see in a few minutes, the eating strategy is so simple that you could start the program tomorrow.

That fact is what partially attracted Dr. Taylor to his approach, and the results are reflected in the decade-long research performed in his New Castle University imaging lab.

In 2011, Dr. Taylor published the first of several studies using an energy-restricted therapeutic diet for a group of patients with type-2 diabetes. At the end of just eight weeks, the participants, on average, dropped their HbA1c from 7.4 percent to 6.0 percent, lost twenty-nine pounds, and reduced their fasting insulin levels by almost 60 percent.[147]

Furthermore, in the test group, liver fat was reduced by 70 percent and pancreatic fat by almost 25 percent. At the end of the study, patients' levels of organ fat were similar to those of the non-diabetic control group.

The majority of the patients were also told to discontinue their diabetes medications.

In his conclusion to the study, Dr. Taylor stated, "Normalization of both beta-cell function and hepatic insulin sensitivity in type-2 diabetes was achieved by dietary energy restriction alone."

In 2018, in the journal *Lancet*, Dr. Taylor published the results of another study called the DiRECT Trial, with equally impressive results. In this study, over 300 patients from forty-nine primary care practices in Scotland and England participated in his program. Of the treatment group, almost half (46 percent) achieved remission of type-2 diabetes, eliminating diabetes medications.[148]

THE CASE FOR FAST CHANGES

There's a common notion that "slow and steady wins the race." But is this true?

According to the majority of the medical literature available, the answer is no. Interestingly, it's just the opposite. The faster the weight loss and blood sugar changes, the better the long-term results will be.

This fact was demonstrated in Dr. Taylor's research, as most of the significant changes happened within the first few weeks of the study. After that, the participants continued to improve but much more slowly.

One study, published in the *International Society of Behavioral Medicine* journal, pointed out that in a group of middle-aged, obese women, "Fast weight losers obtained greater weight reduction and long-term maintenance and were not more susceptible to weight regain than gradual weight losers."[149]

Another study in the journal *Obesity Reviews* found that "a greater initial weight loss as the first step of a weight management program may result in improved sustained weight maintenance."[150]

In other words, the faster the weight loss changes, the better the results will be, and the higher likelihood that they will be maintained over time.

These findings fly in the face of the long-held notion that it's better to make changes slowly and gradually, cutting a few hundred calories per day from the diet or getting a few more steps each day.

As described in a paper published in the *New England Journal of Medicine*, called "Myths, Presumptions, and Facts about Obesity," this is one of the most widely held myths. As they explained: "Passionate interests, the human tendency to seek explanations for observed phenomena, and everyday experience appear to contribute to strong convictions about obesity, despite the absence of supporting data."[151]

HOW DOES THE PROFAST DIET WORK?

I mentioned earlier in this chapter that this program was simple, and it is.

I did not say it was easy, and it's not.

The ProFAST diet is for highly motivated people to get their blood sugar down, lose the stubborn fat around their midsection, and eliminate diabetes medications.

It involves an energy-restricted diet of around 600–800 calories per day, prioritizing protein from high-quality sources such as lean beef, chicken, turkey, fish, seafood, and eggs.

In addition to the protein, you'll be eating fibrous vegetables such as leafy greens, broccoli, cauliflower, and salads with a minimal amount of fats and oils.

What you won't be eating is fruits, nuts, fatty cuts of meat, avocado, coconut, beans, grains, and sugars.

Sound limited? It is.

Fortunately, there are ways to make it more interesting with spices, marinades, salad dressings, and some creativity. We've included fifty recipes in the back of the book to help you navigate the eating plan without losing your mind.

Here's the question you might want to ask yourself: "Am I willing to follow a restrictive, limited eating plan for six weeks so that I can thoroughly enjoy the rest of my life?"

FOOD AS FUEL, NOT AS ENTERTAINMENT

There are many reasons people eat. We eat for fun, for comfort, to distract us from pain, because we are bored or stressed, or because we are addicted to certain foods. There is really only one reason that we should be eating: nourishment.

There are many other ways to entertain yourself. Pick up a new hobby. Go for a walk. Spend some time with your spouse or your family. Travel to somewhere you've never been. Read a good book. Just don't make food your source of entertainment.

Don't get me wrong; you can enjoy your food. But if you have diabetes and blood sugar problems, it helps if you're not eating to entertain or medicate yourself.

This program is not a long-term eating strategy. I'll discuss the maintenance eating recommendations later in this book. the ProFAST diet is a short-term, therapeutic tool to help you overcome the insulin resistance associated with diabetes by melting the fat stored in your liver and around your organs.

If you're still with me, here are some details of what you'll be doing during the three phases of the ProFAST diet.

PHASE I: PREPARATION

Amelia Earhart is credited with stating, "Preparation, I have often said, is rightly two-thirds of any venture." Just in case that's true, it's essential to take the time to prepare for what lies ahead.

The first two weeks of the ProFAST diet are dedicated to preparation, and there are a few supplies that you'll need.

SUPPLEMENTS

As part of the program, it's essential to use a few supplements. These are not optional. I'll discuss these nutrients in detail later in this book, but you'll want to make sure you have them ahead of time.

The most critical supplements include:

- High-quality, organic multivitamin, multi-mineral supplement
- DHA- and EPA-rich purified fish oil product
- Electrolyte product containing magnesium, sodium, potassium, and chloride

A good-quality supplemental fiber product can also be beneficial.

After multiple requests, I designed several products specifically for this program. It's called The ProFAST Bundle and is available at sweetlifenutritionals.com.

RECIPES AND MEAL PLAN

As I mentioned earlier, during this program, while you should certainly enjoy your food, you'll be focusing on food as fuel rather than entertainment. Find a few recipes that you like, and build your meal plan in advance so you're not stuck with no idea what to eat.

YOUR DIET AND PHYSIOLOGY

The ProFAST diet will be much easier if you are already burning fat as your primary fuel source and you are not addicted to sugar.

During the first two weeks, we recommend that you follow a low-carbohydrate diet, focusing on eating less than 100 grams of carbohydrates per day. You can then start incorporating more protein into your diet, and there's no need to restrict healthy fats.

This strategy will prime the pump for fat burning and help your cells be less dependent on dietary sugar and carbohydrates.

Feel free to snack during this phase, if necessary, to stay on track and prevent excessive hunger.

MINDSET

Lastly, and most importantly, you'll want to get your mind right for the coming weeks. Prepare yourself mentally by focusing on what's important to you—on why you want to get your blood sugar down and beat diabetes.

Start by writing down your three to five most important goals for the next six weeks. Ask yourself why you want to get these results and what your life will look like once you get there.

Then, think about what obstacles will likely get in your way. Perhaps you'll find yourself at a friend's home with no good food options or find yourself wanting to eat at night. Solve these problems ahead of time. Decide now how you'll overcome your obstacles.

When you already have the solution in your back pocket, you're much less likely to veer off track from foreseeable challenges.

Finally, write a statement of commitment. Here's an example:

> "I commit to my health and myself by working on reducing body fat and blood sugar by getting regular physical activity, monitoring my food intake, and eating foods consistent with my long-term goals to reverse diabetes, while staying positive and enjoying this process of becoming a healthier version of myself."

Write a statement that is true for you and inspires you to renew your commitment to follow your plan each morning.

PHASE II: ENGAGEMENT

Once you've taken the time to get your mind right, prime your fat-burning pump, create your personalized meal plan, and stock up on your supplements, it's time to engage in the Pro-FAST diet.

The engagement phase lasts for up to six weeks, and there are several levels of intensity that you can choose based on your weight, body-fat percentage, blood sugar, and commitment.

I'll outline the program in detail in the next chapter.

PHASE III: TRANSITION

After you've spent six weeks engaging in the ProFAST diet, losing weight, reducing your blood sugar and lipids, and transforming your body and health, it's time to lock in the changes.

One of the biggest problems with losing weight and reducing fat mass is that most people will regain some fat once they go back to regular eating. Even in most studies done using the protein-sparing modified fast, the participants regain most of the weight they lost by five years.

Understanding how and why this happens and creating a strategy to overcome this phenomenon is the key to long-term change and diabetes reversal.

Later, I'll discuss how to reprogram your homeostatic set point to maintain weight loss and blood sugar changes.

OLLIE'S TRANSFORMATION

As I was preparing to write this book, I stumbled upon an article in *Women's World* magazine called, "How One Mom Lost Half Her Weight on a Fat-Melting Diet Normally Used by Body Builders." Needless to say, it got my attention.[152]

It was about a woman named Ollie, who, at 345 pounds, was

scared for her life and the future of her son and was considering bypass surgery. She went to the Cleveland Clinic, where her doctor recommended a protein-sparing modified fast program. After years of frustration and with her health on the line, the medically supervised, aggressive program felt like her only option.

The story goes on to share how, after eighty days, Ollie hit fifty pounds lost and "did a happy dance." But she didn't stop there. Another year later, she had lost 185 pounds and transformed her life.

Describing her experience, she said, "I've had to work a little harder than most to live a 'normal' life, but the rewards are worth it."

Let's take a closer look at how the ProFAST diet works and precisely what you'll be eating.

CHAPTER 8

IMPLEMENTING THE PROFAST DIET

Sandra came to see me in my office after struggling with her weight for years. In addition to type-2 diabetes, she was dealing with an imbalance in thyroid hormones from a condition called Hashimoto's thyroiditis. Hashimoto's is an autoimmune disease that attacks the thyroid, leaving the body with low thyroid hormone levels. She had been medicated with a synthetic thyroid hormone, which helped her energy, but she still couldn't lose weight. Sandy told me that she gained weight just looking at food.

When she came to me, she was frustrated with how she looked and felt, her blood sugar levels and weight, and the medications she had to take every day. She didn't want more pills—she wanted to fix the problem.

After working together for two months with minimal results, I mentioned the ProFAST diet to her and asked if she'd be willing to give it a try. "I'll do just about anything if it works," she told me. So I explained the program to her, and off she went.

Five days later, Sandy called my office. My assistant said to me, "Doc, you're going to want to hear this!"

When I got on the phone, Sandy said to me, "I can't believe it, but this actually works!" She explained how she had already lost six pounds, that her pants were looser, and she felt better than she could ever remember.

Sandy continued on the plan for another seven weeks, losing a total of eighteen pounds and finally getting her blood sugar into the normal range.

THE PROFAST FOOD PLAN

The ProFAST diet is first and foremost about real food. This program is not a liquid calorie diet or a regimen where you'll be encouraged to eat processed foods laced with preservatives and artificial sweeteners. You'll be eating real, whole food—just less of it.

The program is based on the highest nutrient density foods available, with the best protein-to-energy ratio using lean proteins and fibrous, non-starchy vegetables. In addition to these, you can use herbs, spices, seasonings, and minimal amounts of fruits and added oils.

PROTEIN CHOICES

The ProFAST diet is not technically a fast. On the contrary, you'll be eating a wide variety of healthy protein-rich foods and lots of fibrous vegetables. The fats in your diet will come mostly from protein-centric foods with minimal added oils.

Fish

Fish is a wonderful source of protein and nutrition, including fat-soluble vitamins and omega-3 fatty acids. It's considered an incredibly heart-healthy food, with multiple studies showing a reduction in heart attacks, strokes, and other cardiovascular diseases with fish consumption.[153]

Most white fish are exceptionally lean with a protein-to-energy ratio of up to 7:1, so eating fish is a great way to minimize fat consumption. This quality will allow you to burn more of your body fat.

Darker fish, like salmon, while higher in fat, contains large amounts of essential omega-3 fatty acids, such as DHA and EPA. These omega-3 fats have been shown to improve brain and eye health, reduce inflammation, and lower cholesterol and triglyceride levels.[154]

Eating fish regularly has been associated with having a bigger and better brain, leading to less depression and better sleep.[155]

One concern with fish is the amount of mercury and other contaminants from polluted oceans. While this is undoubtedly a concern, the fish with the highest mercury levels are at the top of the food chain and include shark, marlin, tuna, swordfish, king mackerel, and tilefish.

GOOD SOURCES OF LEAN FISH INCLUDE:

- Cod
- Haddock
- Flounder
- Halibut
- Tilapia
- Pollock
- Orange roughy

Salmon can be eaten once per week for a boost of omega-3 fats. While smaller fish like herring, sardines, and mackerel are excellent sources of omega-3 fatty acids, they are too high in overall fat for the ProFAST diet.

Shellfish

One of the best sources of lean protein is nutrient-rich shellfish. Most shellfish carry between a 4:1 and a whopping 10:1 protein-to-energy ratio, making them perfect additions for the ProFAST diet.

The fats contained in shellfish are mainly omega-3 fatty acids necessary for cell membrane health, lipid control, and brain and eye health and to reduce inflammation.

Many shellfish are power-packed with nutrients, such as zinc, magnesium, iron, and vitamin B12.

Shellfish consumption is cardioprotective. One study, published in the *American Journal of Epidemiology,* found that men who consumed more shellfish had less chance of having a heart attack and a 20 percent decrease in overall death rate.[156]

The only drawback with shellfish is that some sources contain contaminants such as cadmium and mercury. However, studies show that they have less mercury than the larger fish at the top of the food chain.

Lean Beef

Lean beef is one of the best sources of complete protein and contains a wide variety of essential micronutrients. For the ProFAST diet, we recommend 90/10 beef, which means that it contains only 10 percent fat. This percentage yields a protein-to-energy ratio of almost 3:1.

High-quality beef is a valuable source of conjugated linoleic acid (CLA), which has been shown to increase fat burning and weight loss. Beef is unique because it contains some elusive compounds like creatinine, taurine, and glutathione, which provide energy and antioxidant support. It also has iron, selenium, zinc, phosphorus, and B vitamins like B12 and niacin.

Beef has been shown to prevent anemia, increase lean muscle mass, improve exercise performance, and boost energy levels.[157]

I recommend using grass-fed beef, which tends to be less contaminated and has a better fatty acid profile, with a higher concentration of omega-3 fats. Grass-fed beef also has more vitamin E, antioxidants, and CLA and less overall fat.

Bison

Bison comes from American buffalo and is an excellent, naturally lean source of high-quality protein. Like beef, bison is an excellent source of iron, zinc, and a host of other essential micronutrients, and it's naturally lower in fat, which makes it perfect for the ProFAST diet.

Unlike most cattle, bison are more commonly pasture-raised, so most bison meat is naturally grass-fed. So if you're not sure of which meat to choose, bison may be a safer bet.

Chicken and Turkey

Chicken is the go-to protein source for many people. It's naturally lower in fat than beef, so it's also a good fit for the ProFAST diet. In addition to good-quality protein, both chicken and turkey can also be good sources of zinc, iron, selenium, and B vitamins.

If you're going to eat chicken and turkey, you need to be strategic about which part of the bird you eat. The breast is the best fit for this program because it's high in protein and low in fat, with a protein-to-energy ratio of over 8:1. Chicken and turkey legs, including the thigh and drumstick, are still okay in moderation. They provide more micronutrients and yield over twenty grams of protein per serving, with a 2:1 ratio.

Consider using the darker meats occasionally to boost micronutrient levels, and eat the white meats more often for a better protein punch.

It's best, whenever possible, to eat free-range organic turkey and chicken. Conventionally raised chickens are jammed into dirty cages and pumped with antibiotics and growth hormones, which may bioaccumulate in the animal. While not a guarantee of better quality, free-range birds are more likely to be raised healthier.

Pork

Pork from domestic pigs is the most widely consumed "red" meat in the world. It's a nutrient-rich food and a great source of quality, lean protein.

Lean pork loin has many of the same qualities as beef, including being a good source of micronutrients and beneficial compounds like CLA, glutathione, and creatinine. Pork also contains thiamine, magnesium, and potassium.

Pork is higher in oleic acid, which is the monounsaturated fat associated with the Mediterranean diet and olive oil. It also has more omega-3 fats than beef.

Avoid bacon, sausage, ham, and other processed pork products. These are associated with higher disease risk due to N-nitroso compounds. Because some of these are much higher in fat, they are not supported on the ProFAST diet.

One downside of pork is that most conventionally raised pigs are given excessive antibiotics to prevent infection. Whenever possible, choose organic pork to minimize the risk of antibiotic contamination.

Eggs

Natural eggs, from organically raised, pastured chickens, may be the most perfect superfood. They contain potent antioxidants, carotenoids, and other healthy compounds and are a great source of high-quality, slow-release protein.

Eggs contain lots of micronutrients, including vitamin A, selenium, calcium, iron, potassium, zinc, manganese, vitamin E, and B vitamins such as B12, B2, B5, and folate. They are also a great source of choline, which is vital for brain function, and carotenoids like zeaxanthin and lutein, which protect the eyes.

In contrast to what many people believe, eggs have been shown in clinical research to improve cholesterol profiles by raising HDL and reducing heart disease risk.[158]

Eggs have a high satiety score, so they also make you feel full. One study[159] evaluated eggs in relation to weight loss and found that eating eggs led to a 65 percent greater reduction in body weight, with 16 percent more fat loss, and a 61 percent greater reduction in BMI compared to a meal high in carbohydrates.

Since whole eggs have a 1:1 protein-to-energy ratio, we recommend eating one yolk for every two egg whites to increase the ratio.

Vegetarian Protein Sources

As I mentioned earlier in the book, I've worked with many clients who choose to eat a plant-based diet and still want to follow the ProFAST diet. While animal-based protein sources are generally known to be of higher quality due to their composition of amino acids and greater bioavailability, there are several good vegetarian sources of protein.

Fat-Free Cottage Cheese

Cottage cheese is one of the easiest ways to get high-quality lean protein with a high protein-to-energy ratio. It's also a great source of calcium and contains sodium, which can be helpful during the ProFAST diet. It also contains B vitamins like B12, B3, B6, and folate, as well as zinc, copper, and choline.

Studies show that cottage cheese provides the same feeling of fullness as eggs, with less fat and a better protein-to-energy ratio.[160]

Cottage cheese is high in casein, one of the dominant proteins in dairy products, a slow-releasing protein. This characteristic leads to increased satiety from cottage cheese and benefits with maintenance and growth of lean body mass.

Low-Fat Plain Greek Yogurt

Greek yogurt is much higher in protein than regular yogurt and comes in varieties that are also low in fat and carbohydrates. It's also an excellent source of calcium, iodine, and vitamin B12, and it contains natural probiotic strains to boost your gut microbiome.

Studies show that Greek yogurt can lower blood pressure, increase lean muscle mass, build gut health, and reduce feelings of stress, depression, and anxiety.[161]

An analysis of the Women's Health Initiative, looking at over 82,000 post-menopausal women, found that the women who ate more yogurt had a decreased risk of type-2 diabetes. The association did not hold up for other dairy products.[162]

One of my favorite Greek yogurt products is called Two Good. It has an almost 3:1 protein-to-energy ratio with twelve grams of protein per serving.

Whole Soy: Tofu, Tempeh, Edamame

Soy is one of the most versatile and complete plant protein sources available. Although not as balanced as animal protein, it contains all nine essential amino acids and comes in a variety of incarnations.

Tofu is essentially soybean curd, compressed in a way similar to cheese. It comes in a variety of textures from extra firm to silken, similar to soft cheese. While tofu lacks a distinctive taste of its own, it easily absorbs the flavor of whatever it's in, so it tends to be easy to include in meals to give a nice boost of protein.

Tempeh has a more noticeable nutty or earthy flavor and has a firmer, more cake-like texture. Because tempeh is made from fermented soybeans, some people find it easier to digest and prefer it to tofu.

Edamame are young soybeans high in protein, fiber, and other nutrients such as iron, calcium, folate, and vitamin K. They are also an excellent plant source of omega-3 fat.

Consuming high-quality soy protein has been shown to reduce the overall risk of heart disease, reduce hot flashes in perimenopausal women, and reduce the risk of certain hormone-related cancers.[163]

Nutritional Yeast

While it may sound strange to eat yeast, this deactivated *S. cerevisiae* species is a nutrition powerhouse. Nutritional yeast has a mild, cheese-like flavor and is packed with protein, fiber, and nutrients such as zinc, magnesium, copper, manganese, and all the B vitamins, including B12 (when fortified).

Add a few tablespoons of nutritional yeast to your salads or vegetables to increase protein and give them a flavor boost.

Spirulina and Chlorella

Spirulina and chlorella are different types of blue-green algae that are high in protein and loaded with phytonutrients. In addition to protein, spirulina contains potassium, magnesium, manganese, and riboflavin and a powerful antioxidant called phycocyanin, which has shown anti-inflammatory and cancer-protective benefits.[164]

Chlorella might be even better. In addition to being 50–60 percent protein by weight, chlorella is packed with fiber, omega-3 fats, calcium, copper, potassium, folate, vitamin C, iron, and vitamin B12. It's been shown to aid in detoxification by binding toxins, improve lipid levels, reduce blood sugar and blood pressure, and enhance immune function.[165]

Peanut Powder

Powdered peanut butter may seem like a strange concoction made for astronauts, but it's a good fit for the ProFAST diet for people who love the taste of nuts.

In powdered peanut butter, most of the fat is removed from the peanut butter, leaving a lower-calorie product high in fiber and protein. This quality yields a product that has a 2:1 protein-to-energy ratio.

It can be added to a smoothie, sprinkled on a salad, or reconstituted with a little water to make a dip for celery or other vegetables.

My favorite product is called Naked PB, which contains only roasted peanuts and no added sugar.

Complete Plant-Based Protein Powder

Getting ample protein for the ProFAST diet as a vegan can be challenging without adding foods that are also high in carbo-hydrates or fat. One shortcut way to boost protein is by adding a high-quality, plant-based protein product.

There are several inexpensive plant protein powders on the market, including ones made from soy, pea, rice, hemp, and oats. In a pinch, these are better than nothing but not recommended long term as they each have significant drawbacks.

If you choose to use plant-based protein powder, it is best to find a professional-grade, soy-free, blended protein powder that provides a complete protein source with balanced amounts of all nine amino acids.

After searching for the optimal product for years, we were able to create a product called Plant-Powered Protein, which pro-vides seventeen grams of high quality, organic, blended protein with no added flavorings or sweeteners.

To learn more about this product, visit sweetlifenutrionals.com.

VEGETABLES

Fibrous vegetables are the ultimate nutrient-dense food. They are packed with micronutrients, with very few calories and an abundance of naturally filtered water. One of the few consensus areas in nutritional science is fibrous vegetables should be the cornerstone of a healthy diet, and they are included as a significant part of the ProFAST diet

Leafy Green Veggies

These superfoods are packed with nutrients like vitamins A, C, E, and K; iron; manganese; potassium; B vitamins such as riboflavin and folate, antioxidants, carotenoids like beta-carotene and lutein; and other potent phytonutrients.

Several studies have shown cardioprotective benefits of leafy greens and a reduction in risk for type-2 diabetes, cognitive impairment, and various forms of cancer in those who consume certain green vegetables.

SOME OF THE BEST LEAFY GREEN VEGETABLES INCLUDE:

- Spinach
- Kale
- Collard greens
- Watercress
- Cabbage
- Beet greens
- Swiss chard
- Arugula
- Endive
- Turnip greens
- Microgreens

Cruciferous Vegetables

Cruciferous vegetables, named for the cross-like appearance of their blossoms, have long been cherished for their detoxification and chemo-protective benefits. They are high in fiber and extremely nutrient dense.

One thing that distinguishes cruciferous vegetables from others is the presence of a compound called glucosinolates. These powerful phytochemicals have been shown to enhance liver detoxification, protect DNA from damage, reduce cancer-causing agents, and strengthen the immune response to bacteria and viruses.

THESE POWERHOUSE VEGGIES INCLUDE:

- Broccoli
- Cauliflower
- Cabbage
- Kale
- Arugula
- Brussels sprouts
- Turnips
- Radish
- Bok choy

Other Super Veggies

Many other fibrous, high-water-content vegetables are loaded with phytonutrients and low in energy, making them perfect companions to the protein on the ProFAST diet.

THESE SUPER VEGGIES INCLUDE:

- Asparagus
- Celery
- Cucumber
- Garlic
- Ginger
- Sprouts
- Mushrooms
- Onions
- Zucchini
- Eggplant
- Peppers
- Turnips
- Tomatoes (limit)

FRUITS

While fruits are considered healthy by most dietitians and nutritionists, many fruits are high in sugar and carbohydrates compared to the low amount of protein they contain. Most fruit is low in energy (calories) but generally has a poor protein-to-energy ratio, which makes it less than optimal on the ProFAST diet. There are a few exceptions, which are described below.

Berries

Berries, including strawberries, raspberries, blueberries, and blackberries, are among the lowest glycemic and most nutrient dense fruits available. They contain unique phytochemicals, such as anthocyanins, ellagic acid, and resveratrol, which have been shown to protect cells from oxidative damage and decrease disease risk.[166] Berries are also packed with fiber, vitamins, and minerals, such as vitamin C, K1, folate, manganese, and copper.

Several studies have shown that the polyphenols in berries

reduce high blood sugar levels and increase insulin sensitivity, slashing blood insulin levels.[167] They've also been shown to reduce cholesterol levels and inflammation.[168]

Grapefruit

Technically, grapefruit does not fit into the ProFAST diet. However, as a treat in limited moderation, you may find it useful. Grapefruits are packed with vitamins and minerals, and research has shown that grapefruits have a suppressing effect on appetite, reduce insulin levels, increase insulin sensitivity, reduce lipids, and prevent kidney stone formation.[169]

Since they have eleven grams of net carbs and almost no protein, eat them with your other food, and limit yourself to half a grapefruit every few days.

Lemon or Lime

Lemons and limes are low-glycemic, nutrient-dense fruits. They are high in vitamin C and citric acid, which can prevent the accumulation of uric acid and kidney stones, sometimes associated with higher protein intake.[170]

Adding fresh lemon to water may decrease appetite and increase weight loss. Certain compounds in lemons, such as hesperidin and diosmin, have been shown to lower cholesterol and high lipids.[171]

SEASONINGS

Herbs, spices, seasonings, and certain condiments can make your meals much more exciting and help you look forward to eating. If you like these, be sure to include them in your food preparation to add flavor and extra nutrition.

> **HERE ARE SOME OF THE BEST SEASONINGS TO CONSIDER USING:**
>
> - Red chili powder
> - Fresh ground black pepper
> - Real salt or Himalayan salt
> - Fresh herbs such as mint, rosemary, basil, dill, and thyme
> - Vinegar—red, white, and apple cider vinegar
> - Mustard
> - Spices such as cumin, turmeric, cinnamon, and coriander
> - Natural sweeteners such as stevia, monk fruit extract, and allulose

SALAD DRESSINGS AND SAUCES

There are so many commercial salad dressings and sauces available that it is impossible to comment on them in general terms. The best advice is to check the labels.

If they are low in fat and carbohydrate and can fit into your macros (described in the next chapter) without blowing the plan, feel free to use them sparingly.

Some examples of acceptable dressings and sauces include Trader Joe's Green Goddess dressing, which has just two grams of fat and one gram of carbohydrate, and Truff Hot Sauce, which has almost no carbs or fat at all.

FOODS TO AVOID

Many foods should be avoided on the ProFAST diet for obvious and perhaps not-so-obvious reasons. The most important factor for inclusion in the program is that the foods are real, nutrient dense, and have an exceptional protein-to-energy ratio to prioritize protein and decrease energy consumption. Likewise, foods that are packaged, highly processed and refined, or filled with artificial dyes, chemicals, and sweeteners should be avoided, as should those with a high energy-to-protein balance.

EVERYTHING ELSE (SORT OF)

Let me take just a minute to remind you that this is not a forever eating strategy. It's a therapeutic plan designed to supercharge your body to burn fat in your liver and around your organs, improve insulin sensitivity, and reduce blood sugar and blood insulin levels. It can also help you lose weight while maintaining important lean body mass to help you reverse type-2 diabetes.

Some of these foods will be reintroduced during the third phase of the program and can certainly be enjoyed during the long-term maintenance eating plan. During the engagement phase, however, they need to be eliminated.

**HERE IS A LIST OF THE FOODS THAT
YOU'LL NEED TO AVOID FOR A WHILE:**

- Whole and refined grains. This category includes bread, pasta, cereals, oatmeal, rice, quinoa, buckwheat, corn, and everything made with grain-based flours.
- Processed, refined, and natural sugars. These foods include white sugar, brown sugar, cane sugar, honey, coconut palm sugar, agave nectar, and other calorie-containing sugars.
- Beans and legumes (most). The legumes include all beans except soy, such as lentils, black beans, kidney beans, and chickpeas.
- Starchy and sugary vegetables. These foods include starchy vegetables such as sweet potato, white potato, parsnips, green peas, and winter squash and sugary vegetables such as beets and carrots.
- Nuts and seeds. This group includes all nuts and seeds, such as almonds, peanuts, chia, flax, and walnuts.
- Fruits (most). This category includes moderate- and high-glycemic fruits such as apples, pears, most citrus fruits, and tropical fruits and high-fat fruits, such as avocado, coconut, and olives.
- High-fat animal products. These foods include bacon, some beef, chicken wings, and most cheese.
- Added fats and oils. These products include all refined oils such as olive oil, coconut oil, butter, and other seed oils.
- Processed foods and chemical additives. This category includes packaged foods with preservatives, such as bacon, ham, deli meats, and many types of beef jerky and artificial sweeteners (does not include stevia, monk fruit extract, allulose, or erythritol).
- Alcohol. The problem with alcohol is that it stops you from burning fat in your liver. If you want to drink, keep it to a maximum of one serving per day of dry wine or one ounce of pure spirits. Realize that this may interfere with your progress or slow your results.

DRINKS

Much like food, the beverage selection on the ProFAST diet is simple and straightforward. The most important rule to remember is not to drink your calories. We want to save our energy input for the foods in the diet rather than wasting them on drinks.

Filtered or Spring Water

It's important to stay well hydrated during the ProFAST diet. We recommend drinking one ounce of water per kilogram of body weight, up to 80 ounces per day, and no less than sixty-four ounces per day. Water is essential to prevent dehydration, support kidney function, and help flush toxins from the body.

Sparkling Water

If you're looking for something more interesting to drink, consider adding some sparkling water. You can use the classic Perrier or try one of the many new no-calorie, no-sweetener sparkling water products like La Croix or Bubly. These products add more acidity to the body, so I don't recommend more than twenty-four ounces per day.

Coffee

If you're a coffee fan, you'll be happy to know that black coffee and espresso are acceptable and encouraged in the ProFAST diet. Coffee contains antioxidants and chlorogenic acids, which are potent polyphenols. It's also a source of micronutrients such as manganese, magnesium, and specific B vitamins. Caffeine (also found in green and black tea) has been shown to increase fat oxidation and improve energy, mood, and cognitive function.[172]

Multiple studies have shown that coffee drinkers have much lower rates of type-2 diabetes and Alzheimer's disease.[173]

Black, Green, and Herbal Tea

Black and green tea, including matcha tea, are excellent sources of plant polyphenols and antioxidants. One such catechin, called EGCG, has been shown to protect cells from oxidative stress, boost energy, and increase fat burning.[174]

One study published in the *Annals of Internal Medicine* showed that people who drank the most green tea had a 42 percent lower risk of developing type-2 diabetes.[175]

Herbal teas can also be enjoyable, and many carry medicinal properties, supporting mental and physical health.

Almond Milk

While regular or low-fat cow's milk is not recommended on the ProFAST diet due to the sugar content, unsweetened almond milk is acceptable in moderation.

Consider Using a Superfood Powder

Some people like to add superfood powders to their water or almond milk. These are an excellent way to boost micronutrients in the diet without adding substantial energy in the form of carbohydrates or fat.

We created a high-quality, professional product from gently dehydrated organic fruits and vegetables, removing sugar and oils, which leaves a powerful blend of superfood nutrients.

To learn more about the SweetLife Superfood Blend, visit sweetlifenutritionals.com.

WHEN CAN I EAT?

As described in the chapter on fasting, there are numerous benefits to using a restricted eating window throughout the day, week, or month. By staying in a fasted state longer, you'll minimize insulin output, improve leptin sensitivity, and stimulate ketogenesis, which helps reduce inflammation and suppresses appetite.

During the ProFAST diet, you can eat two to three times per day within a restricted eating window. This time frame should be no more than twelve hours, and most people find that they do better with a six- to ten-hour eating window.

A twelve-hour eating window could be eight o'clock in the morning to eight o'clock in the evening, and a six-hour eating window might be noon to six o'clock in the evening. This timing can vary from day to day and is mainly dependent upon your goals, lifestyle, and eating preferences. For example, some people find it challenging to get their daily protein supplies during two meals in a six-hour window. In this case, you can expand the window and eat more times if necessary.

The important thing is to give your body as long as possible without food every twenty-four hours to deplete glycogen storage in the liver and burn stored body fat around the organs and subcutaneous tissue.

CHOOSE YOUR PATH

The ProFAST diet is an intense energy-restriction eating program designed to burn massive amounts of stored body fat while sparing muscle and lean body mass. Whichever path you choose, this program is not easy, and it's not designed to be a long-term strategy. That said, many people find this program to be liberating. Once they get acquainted with the daily schedule and food choices, they surrender to the plan and find that the structure and simplicity make it superior to other strategies.

There are three paths of varying intensity that you can choose based on your starting point and your goals.

Level 1: Moderate

The moderate plan is for people looking for significant changes in body fat loss and blood sugar reduction at a steady pace. This path is typically for men with an estimated body fat percentage of greater than 15 percent and women with an estimated body fat percentage of greater than 20 percent.

Level 2: Accelerated

The accelerated plan is for people looking for deeper body fatness changes and who need to lower blood sugar levels and reduce insulin resistance significantly. This path is typically for men with an estimated body fat percentage of greater than 20 percent and women with an estimated body fat percentage of greater than 25 percent.

Level 3: Aggressive

The aggressive plan is for people looking for major changes in body fatness, blood sugar levels, and insulin sensitivity and those who want to reverse pre-diabetes or type-2 diabetes while minimizing the need for diabetes medications. This path is typically for men with an estimated body fat percentage of greater than 25 percent and women with an estimated body fat percentage of greater than 30 percent.

The ProFAST Plan is not recommended for those with type-1 diabetes, men with a body fat percentage of less than 15 percent, or women with a body fat percentage of less than 20 percent.

CALCULATING MACROS (OR NOT)

There are two ways to proceed with the ProFAST diet. The first is for those who want to carefully track their macronutrients to follow the plan to ensure optimal results. The second, which I'll discuss later, is for those who don't like counting and want a simple structure to follow. Either way, I recommend reading and studying this next section carefully.

Start with Protein

When designing your ProFAST diet, it's imperative to start with the most critical nutrient: protein. According to Drs. Stephen Phinney and Jeff Volek, optimal protein consumption to maintain lean body mass is between 1.2 and 2.0 grams of protein per kilogram of "reference weight" or ideal body weight.[176]

Most of the studies on the protein-sparing modified fast, including the protocol used by Drs. Blackburn and Bistrian and more recently at the Cleveland Clinic, use 1.5 grams of protein per kilogram of ideal body weight.[177] Therefore, this is the recommendation for the ProFAST diet.

HOW TO CALCULATE YOUR IDEAL BODY WEIGHT

There are several ways to estimate optimal or ideal body weight. The first is by looking at a BMI chart and choosing a weight between 18.6 and 24.9. This range is broad and may not be very accurate.

The second method is more personalized to you. You base your optimal body weight on yourself at a time when you felt your best and were at what you consider to be your ideal weight. This method is highly subjective, but it is often the most accurate way to estimate your optimal body weight.

The third method involves consulting a chart of "reference weight" used by Drs. Phinney and Volek in their work. This chart can be found in the resource section at profastdiet.com.

When we guide our clients, we use all three methods to create a consensus for estimating ideal or optimal body weight.

After you've estimated your ideal body weight, divide that number by 2.2 for kilograms. Then multiply that number by 1.5. This formula is expressed in the following calculation:

$$\text{Daily protein intake} = (\text{IBW}/2.2) \times 1.5$$

The daily protein intake should be divided evenly by the number of meals that you eat throughout the day.

Carbohydrate and Fat

Now that you have your protein intake calculated, the next step is to figure out how much carbohydrate and fat you should be eating on the ProFAST diet.

This step is where your program intensity level should be considered. Use the following chart to determine your carbohydrate and fat consumption based on your program intensity level:

- Level 1: Moderate—40–50 grams of net carbohydrate, 40–50 grams of fat per day
- Level 2: Accelerated—30–40 grams of net carbohydrate, 30–40 grams of fat per day
- Level 3: Aggressive—20–30 grams of net carbohydrate, 20–30 grams of fat per day

According to Drs. Phinney and Volek, minimum recommended fat consumption is thirty grams per day to prevent gallstones.[178] This number correlates well with a report in the journal *Gastroenterology*, which concluded that less than thirty grams of fat led to complete gallbladder contraction in test subjects.[179]

In a study published in *Nutrition Journal* in 2017, the authors stated that the WHO says that fat consumption should not go below 20 percent of maintenance energy intake to "ensure adequate consumption of total energy, essential fatty acids, and fat-soluble vitamins, and prevent atherogenic dyslipidemia."[180]

Technically, there is no lower limit for carbohydrate consumption. However, we have found that limiting carbohydrates to less than twenty grams per day is too restrictive for most people and negatively impacts nutrient density by significantly limiting vegetable and fiber consumption.

Here's a real-life example to help make this clearer. For someone on the Aggressive path who weighs 180 pounds and has an ideal weight of 130 pounds, here are the macros:

- Protein: 88 grams per day, split between three meals of about 30 grams.
- Carb: 30 grams per day, split between three meals of about 10 grams.

- Fat: 30 grams per day, split between three meals of about 10 grams.

For example, this could be a salad with 3–4 cups of raw spinach, 1/2 chopped tomato, sliced cucumbers, and mushrooms, with two tablespoons of Green Goddess dressing and 4–5 ounces of grilled chicken breast.

> There are several excellent apps for tracking macronutrient consumption, including Keto Diet App, Carb Manager, Fit Day, My Fitness Pal, and Calorie King. Find an app that you like, and log everything you eat to track your success.
>
> Alternatively, you can use the Self Nutrition Database to look up nutrition data for the foods that you are eating. This information can be found at nutritiondata.self.com.

THE SIMPLE PLAN

If you don't want to be bothered by calculating macros and counting your fat and carb grams, you can use the simple plan as an alternative.

You'll still need to make sure you get adequate protein by doing the calculations described above. Once you know how much protein you need, you can fill in the rest of your meal with high-fiber, low-carbohydrate vegetables and minimal fats. Most of the fat you'll be eating will come from your protein sources.

You can look at the recipes in this book for examples of how to construct a variety of meals to fit your preferences without exceeding the guidelines for fat and carbohydrate consumption.

If your weight loss or blood sugar progress stalls, you can always go back and calculate your macros later to make sure you're not overeating.

WHAT ABOUT EXERCISE?

While physical activity and exercise are important in general, they are mostly not recommended during the ProFAST diet. Exercise classes, running or jogging, high-intensity training, and serious weight training will put extra demands on your body and will lead to higher muscle turnover, which may be harmful while on this program.

Instead of a structured exercise program, during the ProFAST diet, it's more important to stay as active as possible. Keep moving throughout the day. Take the stairs instead of the elevator. Play with the kids or grandkids. Or take the dog outside for a walk around the neighborhood.

EASIER THAN YOU THINK

While I've tried to be clear that the ProFAST diet is not a long-term eating strategy and is highly restrictive, some people find the program refreshingly simple to follow.

One of my clients, Robyn, had been on and off every diet available. She had tried low-fat diets, a low-carb paleo diet, the Master Cleanse, a high-fat keto diet, and an intuitive eating strategy. Some of them worked for a while, but nothing she tried had been genuinely effective. She was still obese with progressively higher blood sugar levels and type-2 diabetes, while on multiple diabetes medications.

When she met me, she was struggling with a plant-based vegan diet. Not only was she not losing weight eating lots of fruit, whole grains, and beans, but her blood sugar was going up, and she was bloated and had no energy. It was a total disaster. The vegan doctor she was working with called her a "non-responder" and said he had never seen a case like hers.

Robyn reluctantly started the ProFAST diet, under my supervision, and within two weeks completely turned her life around. She lost ten pounds in those two weeks, broke her sugar and carbohydrate cravings, which were ruling her life, and dropped her blood sugar over 100 mg/dl (it had been running in the low to mid-200s and dropped under 130 mg/dl on average).

The best part, however, is that Robyn was not struggling. She told me that it was easier than anything else she had ever done. She described how she could let go of her addiction to food and follow the simple eating plan without overthinking it.

She remained on the plan for an additional four weeks and continued to get results. Her blood sugar eventually stabilized in the mid-90s, and she lost another twelve pounds in those four weeks for a total of twenty-two pounds.

Like Robyn, you may find that the ProFAST diet is easier than it seems. Once you organize your eating plan and focus on food for nourishment rather than entertainment, you might end up feeling like this is the simplest and best program you've ever followed.

CHAPTER 9

THE KEY TO LASTING CHANGE

In a study performed at the Cleveland Clinic, the authors described the protein-sparing modified fast as "a rigorous way of rapidly losing a large amount of weight."[181] In their study, the average participant lost almost twenty-five pounds and over 10 percent of their body weight.

But in the early days of the protein-sparing modified fast experiments, the focus was on quick weight loss specifically for obese patients who needed a miracle. Their lives depended on it.

The good news is that it works.

In the *Infant, Child, & Adolescent Nutrition Journal*, the authors reported a case study of a seven-year-old Hispanic girl they referred to as "EF." EF was over 240 pounds with a BMI of forty-two when she started on the PSMF protocol. In three months on the PSMF program, she lost over forty pounds, and her BMI dropped to thirty. Her A1c came down from 5.8 percent to 5.3

percent. Her liver enzymes and triglycerides normalized, and her fasting insulin was reduced by 36 percent.[182]

Dr. George Blackburn, who did much of the original research on protein-sparing diets, noted one problem, however, which has since been leveled as the primary critique for the PSMF: the results don't last. In fact, after he helped create the original PSMF programs, he eventually used gastric bypass surgery to help obese patients, performing the first Roux-en-Y gastric bypass procedure in New England in 1973.[183] Most of the patients who used the PSMF would eventually gain back most of the weight that they lost.

This concern is a legitimate challenge and needs to be solved if we are to ensure positive long-term results.

A study published in 2020 found that "in clinical practice, the PSMF achieves rapid weight loss in the first six months, but only a small percentage of patients maintained significant weight loss long term." Compared to the control group that used a variety of other weight loss methods such as "balanced eating," the group that followed the PSMF only achieved a 3 percent greater weight loss at five years.[184] That's not great.

To understand how to solve this problem—to prevent weight gain, create long-term improvements in blood sugar, and stay diabetes-free—we need to discuss how the brain monitors and controls our physiology.

HOW WEIGHT LOSS WORKS

There's a theory in obesity research, called set point theory, which attempts to explain why most participants in weight loss studies will regain the majority of weight they lose. The general idea is that we all have a "normal" body weight, based on genotype (genetics) and phenotype (how our genes get expressed in the body) and that even if you lose weight below that number, you'll eventually regain to match your predetermined shape. Sounds depressing, doesn't it?

Fortunately, many studies have found this theory to be wrong, or at least incomplete.

The truth is that bodyweight is controlled by a wide variety of factors, including genetics, stress levels, sleep quality, environment, hormone balance, psychological factors, and the foods you are eating—including macronutrient and micronutrient levels.[185]

The body indeed wants to maintain dynamic homeostasis, which means that your brain (hypothalamus) will do everything it can to maintain your weight, body temperature, and other essential factors. Your survival largely depends on this consistency.

Research shows that this homeostatic "set point" can be changed over time to represent current weight, fat mass, lean body mass, and energy expenditure. This adjustable balance has been termed the "settling point."[186]

MAKING THE RESULTS STICK

There's no question that the ProFAST diet and other similar low-energy diets such as the original protein-sparing modified fast work. The research is clear that people lose massive amounts of fat while maintaining lean muscle and metabolic rate. So how do we solve the problem of whether those results stick?

In 2017, a research paper was published in the journal *Endocrine Practice* that demonstrated a partial solution.

They found that at the end of the protein-sparing modified fast, if they gave specific "refeeding instructions" to continue to restrict carbohydrates, 61.1 percent of participants were able to maintain their positive changes at twenty-four months, versus just 26.9 percent who did not follow the instructions.[187]

Another article, published in *Nutrition and Diabetes* in 2014, found that a group of patients with type-2 diabetes, pre-diabetes, and normal glucose all lost weight using a program similar to the ProFAST diet and were able to maintain the changes at twelve months with the appropriate refeeding program.[188]

Several other studies have indicated the importance of maintaining optimal protein intake and keeping carbohydrates or glycemic index low, which leads to better outcomes and improved maintenance of weight loss.[189]

Based on the currently available research and our experience working with thousands of clients using the ProFAST diet, we've developed an eating strategy to transition toward a maintenance diet without losing the results that you've worked so hard to achieve.

MAINTENANCE STRATEGIES

It seems that once your body maintains its current weight, body fat, and lean mass for about thirty days, it establishes a new settling point and will work to maintain that new homeostasis. Therefore, once you've completed the six weeks in the engagement phase of the ProFAST diet, you'll start increasing your energy consumption gradually over four weeks.

During week one of the transition phase, we recommend maintaining your protein consumption and carbohydrate restriction and adding only additional energy from fat. You can add some avocado, cook your vegetables in a heat-friendly oil, or sprinkle some nuts on your salad. Typically, the goal will be to increase your fat consumption by 50 percent of what you were eating. So if you were consuming thirty grams of fat, you would increase that to forty-five grams.

During week two of the transition phase, you'll continue to maintain protein consumption while increasing your fat use once again. To include more fat, you can add other protein sources, such as fattier cuts of beef; higher-fat parts of pork, chicken, and fish; and more whole eggs. You can also increase your use of cheese, cream, butter, and other healthy oils. Fat consumption in week two of transition will typically be twice what you were eating during the engagement phase. So if you were originally eating thirty grams of fat, you would increase to a total of sixty grams of fat per day.

In week three of the transition phase, you'll maintain protein levels while moderately increasing your carbohydrate and fat consumption. For carbohydrates, you can increase your intake by up to 25 percent of the amount you were eating on the Pro-FAST diet. If you were eating thirty grams of carbs, you would increase to 37.5 grams. This adjustment means adding some extra fruit, beans, or small amounts of starchy vegetables. For fat, you'll increase up to 150 percent of your intake on the program, without exceeding your maintenance amount (discussed in a coming chapter).

Finally, during week four of transition, you'll be increasing fat consumption up to 200 percent what you were eating on the ProFAST diet and carbohydrates up to 50 percent while maintaining protein intake. As mentioned above, it's wise not to exceed your maintenance amount for fat and carbs as you'll determine within your long-term strategy.

Carbohydrate tolerance varies significantly between people, so it's essential to watch your blood sugar and weight response as you increase your carbs. Some people find it beneficial to keep carbohydrates low, while others will increase their consumption to seventy-five grams of net carbs per day.

I recommend staying on all of the recommended supplements through the transition phase to ensure micronutrient and electrolyte levels remain balanced and healthy.

ADDED ROUNDS AND PROFAST DAYS

If, after completing the ProFAST diet, you have additional weight to lose or have not fully reached your blood sugar and metabolic health goals, you may want to consider another round or two of the ProFAST diet.

While most people notice that the results are slower and less dramatic during subsequent programs, you can gradually reach your long-term goals if you follow the program multiple times. It's best to take an additional thirty days off after the transition phase ends before starting another ProFAST diet.

If, however, you feel that you've reached maximum improvement or don't want to start another ProFAST Ddet in the near future, then you'll want to focus on maintaining the positive changes that you've made.

One strategy that many of our clients have found to be successful for them to maintain the positive changes is to schedule one or two ProFAST Days per week during the transition.

During the ProFAST Day, you'll follow the same eating strategy that you used during the engagement phase of the ProFAST diet. This strategy can help quickly reset the body from unintended weight gain, inflammation, or addictive eating behaviors.

ADDITIONAL RULES FOR THE TRANSITION PHASE

Based on our clinical experience, there are a few things that we do not recommend during the transition phase. These include the following:

- Snacking on nuts. Feel free to add a few nuts or seeds to your meals, but refrain from eating them alone.
- Snacking on high-fat cheeses. It's fine to add a little cheddar or parmesan cheese to an omelet or a salad, but I do not recommend slicing up cheese as a snack.
- Excessive alcohol. If possible, it's best to continue to avoid alcohol consumption. If you want to drink, consider one

glass of dry wine or one serving of pure spirits per day as a maximum.

- Nutrition bars. Packaged "nutrition bars," even well-balanced ones, tend to provide extra food and extra energy that is mostly unnecessary. They are often used as between-meal snacks and typically stimulate appetite more than suppressing it, leading to overeating. Be careful with these bars.

- Packaged, processed, and refined foods. Even though you'll increase your fat and carbohydrate consumption, I strongly suggest that you continue to minimize or avoid packaged and heavily processed foods such as snack products, most jerky, and industrial seed oils (vegetable oils).

- Addictive foods. If you find that you have a particular food, such as roasted nuts or nutrition bars, that you have trouble limiting, it's best to continue to avoid that food through the transition phase.

- Snacking between meals. During the transition phase and into maintenance, I generally recommend against snacking between meals. It's essential to allow your metabolic hormones to reset by giving them four to five hours between meals with no food.

Once you've successfully transitioned from the ProFAST diet, you'll want to follow a long-term, healthy diet that continues to focus on nutrient-dense real food in a way that creates an energy balance and allows you to maintain optimal weight and blood sugar levels.

LONG-TERM RESULTS

While much of the research indicates that many people regain weight after any weight loss program, including the protein-sparing modified fast, a few specific studies have found strategies that help people maintain weight loss and other positive results.[190]

The first important step is to handle the transition properly. The biggest mistake many people make is that they reduce their protein consumption and increase their fat and carbohydrate consumption too quickly. Be sure to follow the transition plan described earlier to protect the changes you've made.

The second key is to incorporate more physical activity into your daily and weekly routine. Staying active and building fitness and lean body mass is an integral part of overall health and blood sugar control. You'll get better long-term results if you can incorporate some physical activity into your program.

We recommend following the SweetLife™ Pyramid, which has three progressive categories of physical activity.

At the base of the pyramid, we recommend getting at least 150 minutes per week of slow, fat-burning cardio to continue to encourage the body to oxidize fat, especially in a fasted state. This movement can consist of walking, running, swimming, playing outside, sports, biking, or cardio machines such as the recumbent bike or elliptical machine.

These workouts can be divided into three sessions of fifty minutes, five sessions of thirty minutes, or any other variation that adds up to at least 150 minutes each week.

The second type of exercise in the SweetLife™ Pyramid is resistance training. Resistance or strength training can consist of bodyweight exercises, weight machines, resistance bands, and free weights. I recommend scheduling twenty to forty minutes for a complete strength training workout two to three times per week or consider doing short "micro-workouts" of five to ten minutes per day.

Micro-workouts are typically bodyweight exercises, such as press-ups, squats, lunges, and arm curls. Instead of an exhaustive thirty- to sixty-minute workout, choose one bodyweight exercise, and perform as many as possible. Then rest for a minute and repeat that two or three times.

Examples of bodyweight exercises that you can do as part of a micro-workout include:

- Air squats
- Walking lunges
- Single-leg balance
- Jump squats
- Push-ups
- Planks
- Tricep dips
- Burpees

A practice of strength or resistance training is critical to build more mitochondria, increase insulin sensitivity, deplete muscle glycogen, lower blood sugar, and increase metabolic rate by creating a higher level of lean body mass.

The third and final exercise strategy on the SweetLife™ Pyramid is interval or sprint training. This strategy involves short bursts of thirty- to sixty-second high-intensity exercise, followed by one minute of rest. You can then repeat that three to ten times based on the degree of intensity. This type of quick "burst training" can be done multiple times per week.

Sprint training or interval training at a high intensity will quickly deplete glycogen stores in the liver and the muscles, forcing your body to refill that glycogen from the glucose in your blood. This state will improve insulin sensitivity and lower your blood sugar while stimulating growth hormone and muscle repair.

For optimal, long-term maintenance of your weight loss and blood sugar, regular physical activity incorporating all three of these techniques is imperative. This activity will allow your cells to become more insulin sensitive and build more lean body mass, which will help you stay fit and diabetes-free.

RESETTING YOUR PROGRESS

Taking one or two days per week to quickly reset your progress can make a substantial difference in your long-term outcomes. I mentioned one ProFast day per week as a way to help people reprogram their set-point during the transition phase, but it can also be used as a way for you to maintain the progress that you've made.

As an alternative, you may want to consider doing a full fast day once per week instead of a ProFast Day. This approach will help your body upregulate autophagy, which will be dramatically increased during a pure water fast. Autophagy is the breakdown of old, damaged tissue in the body to recycle proteins and other cell structures. Absolute water fasting also lowers IGF-1, associated with some forms of cancer and other problems.

RECOVERING FROM A SETBACK

Suppose you happen to have a relapse—you overeat, consume too many carbohydrates, or get off track with your eating and physical activity plan. In that case, it's crucial to get right back in control as quickly as possible.

There's a phenomenon called the WTH effect, which describes the "What the Heck?" feeling when you get off track with your diet and the resulting poor decisions that are often made when this happens. There's a tendency to lose sight of your progress, loosen your inhibitions, and go on a multiple-day binge to satisfy your pent-up desires. This approach will sabotage your long-term progress.

Instead of letting a mistake take you off track, forgive yourself and correct your path quickly. This decisive and affirmative action will prevent setbacks and give you the best chance of lasting results.

FINDING SUPPORT AND ENCOURAGEMENT

One of the biggest challenges with managing type-2 diabetes, high blood sugar, and being overweight is that it's common to feel isolated. People are often embarrassed or feel guilty that they allowed themselves to develop type-2 diabetes or gain substantial weight. The social isolation that often accompanies these feelings is harmful and leads to a higher likelihood of relapse.

Stay connected with friends, family members, coworkers, and people you see at church or in social gatherings so that you don't feel alone.

One of the best ways to connect and get ongoing support from like-minded people is to join the ProFast Community. You can find our interactive Facebook for the program at facebook.com/groups/profast.

IF AT FIRST YOU DON'T SUCCEED

One of my clients, Charlene, has been through the ProFAST diet program twice. Not because she needed to lose an extraordinary amount of weight or monumentally drop her blood sugar levels, and not because the program didn't work for her. Interestingly, that was the problem: it worked almost too well.

The first time Charlene went through ProFAST, she lost twenty-three pounds, and her HbA1c came down to 5.2 percent (from over 7.0 percent). She had fantastic results almost immediately and found the program to be precisely what she needed. Charlene had been battling pre-diabetes and then type-2 diabetes for years and needed a simple, structured plan to help her get results.

The problems started to happen during the summer. She had just completed the engagement phase of the ProFAST diet and was doing well when she left with her family for a two-week beach vacation. A few days into it, a "taste" of her husband's ice cream turned into her own ice cream, pizza, and potato chips.

A few months later, after the summer, Charlene contacted my office, explained what had happened, and went through the ProFast program again. This time, the results stuck. The last time I heard from Charlene, it had been three years since she completed ProFAST, and she was maintaining her blood sugar under 100 mg/dl and had only gained a few pounds back.

She told me that over the years, she would go off her eating plan here and there but that the key was to correct quickly. As long as she got back on track right away, she was able to retain control and maintain all of the incredible changes she made.

In the next chapter, I will share some more information about essential lab tests and other evaluation metrics that will help you track and monitor your progress during the ProFAST diet.

CHAPTER 10

TESTING AND EVALUATION

In 1975, a pathologist named Joseph Kraft published a letter in the journal *Lancet* in response to an article about pre-diabetes in Pima Indians. In his letter, he asserted that specific insulin patterns are "fundamental" in determining the presence of diabetes or pre-diabetes.[191] He made the case that testing insulin should be the earliest diagnostic test for those struggling with blood sugar.

At that time, blood insulin tests were available but were rarely done outside of the research lab. According to Dr. Kraft's work analyzing over 14,300 blood laboratory exams, there are four distinct patterns of insulin secretion following an oral glucose tolerance test.[192] Understanding these patterns and how the body responds to this glucose load, he demonstrated, gives the clinician valuable information to help people find and correct problems with blood sugar and metabolic health.

In 2017, James DiNicolantonio, Catherine Croft, and others published a paper in *Open Heart*. They described insulin testing as the "earliest biomarker for diagnosing pre-diabetes, type-2 diabetes, and cardiovascular risk."[193] They explained in their paper that high blood insulin levels can lead to high blood pressure, obesity, atherosclerosis, damage to blood vessels, brain disorders, and peripheral neuropathy and may even contribute to certain cancers. This report echoed the work of Dr. Gerald Reaven, published as early as 1967.[194]

Surprisingly, and despite the convincing research published by Dr. Kraft and others, the simple fasting insulin test is still rarely used in clinical practice. Ask your doctor to do it, and they will likely look at you with a confused expression, like a dog responding to a high-pitched whistle.

Why? The sad truth is that most physicians are unaware of the science. Drs. Kraft and Reaven's work offers little benefit to pharmaceutical companies, as they mainly focus on high insulin levels, which there are no widely used medications to treat. Additionally, Dr. Reaven suggested using diet and lifestyle as a primary treatment for insulin resistance and hyperinsulinemia. These areas are far outside the conventional doctor's wheelhouse.

Unfortunately, there's a steep cost for this ignorance. There are hundreds of millions of people worldwide, walking around unknowingly with high insulin levels and insulin resistance, doing incalculable damage to their organs, blood vessels, and brain.

Let's look at another example. Scurvy is a devastating disease that leads to bleeding, black, and gangrenous skin and gums. It was so common a few hundred years ago that governments would assume that half their sailors would die from it on any sea voyage.[195]

Eventually, many captains realized that citrus and certain other foods could prevent scurvy and carried them on board their ships. In the early 1900s, ascorbic acid (vitamin C) was discovered, and human dietary studies in the 1960s showed that vitamin C could stop scurvy.[196]

If we didn't know that a lack of vitamin C prevented or cured scurvy, we would still be fighting this disease today (scurvy still exists, but it's rare). Understanding how the body functions and performing lab tests to assess metabolic health can help guide better outcomes.

While I'm not going to provide a comprehensive guide to functional lab testing and evaluation in this book, I want to highlight some of the most important tests to consider before starting the ProFAST diet. These tests will help you assess your metabolic health status and provide objective feedback about positive health changes.

SIMPLE MEASUREMENTS

Before going over the lab tests, I want to discuss a few measurements that are often recommended to evaluate metabolic health.

BMI

BMI, or Body Mass Index, is often recommended as a marker for metabolic health. It represents a person's weight in comparison to their height. According to the CDC, a high BMI can be an "indicator of body fatness." The problem with BMI is that it's based on weight rather than shape or body fat. Therefore, it tends to be wildly inaccurate.

For example, a 220–pound bodybuilder with less than 10 percent body fat will be considered obese, while a petite, 105-pound lean woman may be regarded as grossly underweight. For these reasons, I generally don't recommend using BMI.

WEIGHT SCALE

Due to the same reasons described above, the bathroom scale is generally not an effective way to assess metabolic health. Without considering the lean mass and fat mass of the individual, it's impossible to make an accurate assessment of risk and health status.

The scale can be used as a quick way to assess overall weight loss progress while on the ProFAST diet. Just realize that it has significant limitations. People will often gain lean muscle while consuming more protein and exercising because they are losing fat. This phenomenon is not expressed by looking at the scale and may misrepresent progress and lead to demotivation.

BODY FAT PERCENTAGE

Measuring body fat percentage is helpful when accurate. Unfortunately, many evaluation methods, including bioimpedance scales and skin calipers, are often misinterpreted or inaccurate. The gold standard is considered hydrostatic (underwater) weighing, which is mainly used in research settings. One highly accurate method is called the Bod Pod. It uses displacement technology and has a minimal error rate. Getting a Bod Pod test takes just a few minutes, usually costs less than $50, and is available in many gyms and fitness facilities.

Interestingly, the method I often recommend for a quick and easy estimation of body fat is a simple visual method. If you can't get a Bod Pod test, find an image online that depicts various body fat percentages, and compare yourself in the mirror to these images to get an estimation of your proportions.

WAIST-TO-HEIGHT RATIO

One of the easiest, quickest, and most cost-effective ways to assess metabolic health is the waist-to-height ratio. Numerous studies indicate that waist-to-height ratio is highly correlated to insulin resistance, metabolic syndrome, and risk for type-2 diabetes and is a better indicator for metabolic health than weight or BMI.

To find waist-to-height ratio, measure your waist one inch above your belly button, and divide the number by your height in the same units (inches or centimeters). A waist-to-height ratio of <0.50 is considered healthy, while a number higher than 0.50 is at higher risk for metabolic disease. For optimal metabolic health, the recommended waist-to-height ratio is 0.43–0.52 for men, and 0.42–0.48 for women.

GLUCOSE SELF-MONITORING

Glucose self-monitoring with a glucometer or CGM (continuous glucose monitor) is highly useful for people with diabetes and blood sugar imbalances. It can be a very effective way to evaluate your body's response to various foods, events, exercise, and states of stress.

I generally recommend testing your blood sugar in a fasted state within thirty minutes of awakening as a baseline. Additionally, pre- and post-challenge tests can be done around individual meals and activities to assess blood sugar response.

Normal fasting blood glucose levels when self-monitoring are 76–92 mg/dl and should not increase by greater than 30 mg/dl after meals.

A CGM tests your blood sugar at regular intervals throughout the day and is a powerful tool to assess glycemic response.

According to the FDA, a glucometer must be accurate to within 15–20 percent of the actual (laboratory) reading and is generally about 5 percent higher than venous blood readings taken in the lab.

LAB TESTS

Many people find that simple measurements are enough to provide a good gauge to assess progress while on the ProFAST diet. Since this program is more intensive than a gradual and incremental diet plan, I typically recommend having a full panel of lab tests completed before starting the program.

Specific markers are critical to evaluate when considering the ProFAST diet, including thyroid health status, blood sugar, hemoglobin A1c, minerals and electrolytes, and uric acid. Work with your physician to determine which of these tests would be most valuable for you.

COMPREHENSIVE METABOLIC PANEL

The comprehensive metabolic panel is one of the most common lab tests ordered by physicians and includes a serum glucose, electrolytes, and several markers for kidney and liver function.

Glucose

This is typically done fasting and is considered the standard for diagnosing diabetes and monitoring control and treatment success.

High glucose levels can also be associated with acute stress, prednisone or other steroid treatment, chronic kidney disease, hyperthyroidism, and pancreatitis.

Optimal: 76–92 mg/dl

Lab normal: <100 mg/dl

Pre-diabetes: 100–125 mg/dl

Diabetes: >125 mg/dl (on two exams)

Minerals and Electrolytes

Several minerals are tested as part of a metabolic panel, including calcium, potassium, sodium, and chloride.

Calcium (8.5–10.2 mg/dL) is an essential mineral for bone health and the function of nerves, muscles, and the brain. Too little calcium may be caused by low vitamin D, low parathyroid hormone levels, or a lack of calcium in the diet. In contrast, high calcium is due to hyperparathyroidism, kidney disease, bone disorders, and malignant cancers.

Potassium (3.6–5.2 mmol/L) is an essential electrolyte for nerve and muscle function, including the heart. Too little potassium can cause muscle weakness, cramps, and fatigue, while too much can lead to dangerous heart rhythm problems.

Sodium (135–145 mEq/L) is an electrolyte that allows the body to balance and regulate fluids and is involved with muscle, nerve, kidney, and liver function. Low sodium is usually due to loss of fluid, kidney disease, or low cortisol, aldosterone, or other adrenal hormones. Elevated sodium levels are often due to dehydration but may also be associated with high cortisol.

Chloride (96–106 mEq/L) is another electrolyte that helps to regulate blood pressure. It's also vital for blood pH and blood volume. Elevated levels indicate dehydration and kidney disease and may also be present with acidosis. Low chloride is seen with high cortisol and congestive heart failure.

Kidney Tests

Several necessary kidney tests are done as part of the metabolic panel, including creatinine, BUN, and eGFR. It's also important to check microalbumin in the urine annually.

The kidneys are essential organs for filtering waste from the blood, controlling fluid and mineral levels, and producing certain hormones, red blood cells, and vitamin D.

Creatinine: <1.2 mg/dL women, <1.4 mg/dL men

BUN: 7–20 mg/dL

eGFR: >60

Microalbumin <20 mg/dL

Liver Enzymes

As part of the comprehensive metabolic panel, several tests help detect liver damage or dysfunction. These tests include albumin, ALT, AST, alkaline phosphatase, and GGT.

These proteins and enzymes can be elevated in the presence of damage to tissues such as the lungs, heart, bone, muscles, and liver.

High alkaline phosphatase with high levels of other enzymes indicates liver damage or disease. If the other enzymes are normal, it may indicate bone disease.

High ALT is almost always related to the liver and is the best test to detect hepatitis.

High AST with other elevated enzymes typically indicates a liver problem. In the absence of other elevated enzymes, it may indicate heart or muscle damage.

High GGT is also typically associated with liver disease. This marker has also been associated with increased oxidative stress, metabolic disease, cardiovascular disease, type-2 diabetes, Alzheimer's disease, and cancer.[197] There appears to be a higher risk for these problems as GGT increases above the optimal levels based on gender.

Albumin: 3.5–5.0 g/dL

Alkaline phosphatase: 40–129 U/L

ALT: 7–56 U/L (ideally should be less than 40 U/L)

AST: 10–40 U/L

GGT: 9–48 U/L (optimal for men is <16 U/L and for women is <9 U/L)

Standard Lipid Panel

The standard lipid panel is one of the most controversial lab tests done as part of the recommended testing guidelines. It's part of the ABCs of diabetes, including the monitoring of A1c, blood pressure, and cholesterol, but the implications of high cholesterol have mixed results.

Many physicians will attempt to suppress cholesterol levels, specifically LDL cholesterol, to sub-physiologic ranges using anti-cholesterol agents, such as statin drugs, to prevent heart disease or mitigate the risks of type-2 diabetes. There is little evidence to support this approach.[198]

From a metabolic perspective, several notable patterns may indicate insulin resistance and metabolic dysfunction.

In addition to the basic lipid panel, there are more advanced tests that have shown a stronger correlation to heart disease, such as NMR lipoprotein profile (particle size and count), Lp-PLA2, Apo A-1, Apo B, Lp(a), and remnant lipoprotein.

Total cholesterol: <240 mg/dL is acceptable, <200 mg/dL is considered desirable

HDL cholesterol: >40 mg/dL in men, >50 mg/dL in women

LDL cholesterol: <150 mg/dL is acceptable, <100 mg/dL is considered desirable

Triglycerides: <150 mg/dL is acceptable, <70 mg/dL is optimal

Several ratios are valuable, including:

TC/HDL ratio: <4 is acceptable, <3 is desirable

Trig/HDL ratio: <2 is acceptable, <1 is optimal

Hemoglobin A1c

The hemoglobin A1c test (also called glycated hemoglobin) has become an integral biomarker for monitoring blood sugar control. It measures the percent of glycation of the A1c receptor on the hemoglobin of red blood cells.

This test's significance is that it measures glycation or damage from elevated blood sugar, not the blood sugar itself. Damage in one area, such as the red blood cells, can be correlated to damage in other areas like the blood vessels, kidneys, brain, and other organs.

Research indicates that an A1c above 6.0 percent can potentially lead to pathology from elevated blood sugar or diabetes complications. The higher the A1c, the greater the likelihood of developing complications from elevated blood sugar.

The target range for hemoglobin A1c is hotly debated. Depending on who you ask, you may get two or three different answers for a target goal for the A1c. Here are some ranges that may help clarify the misunderstanding:

Normal hemoglobin A1c: 4.0–5.6 percent

Elevated HbA1c: >5.6 percent

Pre-diabetes: 5.7–6.4 percent

Diabetes: >6.4 percent

AACE recommendation for HbA1c: <6.5 percent

ADA recommendation for HbA1c: <7.0 percent

Fasting Insulin

The fasting insulin test is one of the most useful markers that you can have to evaluate your ability to regulate blood sugar, burn fat, and achieve optimal metabolic health. Unfortunately, most people never get it done.

Insulin is a hormone that helps glucose and amino acids enter your cells, where the glucose gets burned for fuel. When insulin levels are low, you can't properly metabolize glucose, and levels rise. Likewise, when your cells are resistant to insulin, even in the presence of high insulin levels, sugar can't get into the cells to be utilized appropriately.

Additionally, elevated insulin levels (seen in most insulin resistance) damage the lining of your blood vessels, kidneys, nerves, and brain. Insulin is the central "fat storage" hormone in the body, so high insulin levels lead to additional fat storage and block your body's ability to burn fat effectively.

Fasting insulin:

optimal 2.5–6.0 uIU/mL

low <2.0 uIU/mL

moderately high 6.1–10 uIU/mL

high >10 uIU/mL

Insulin Response Test

Like the fasting insulin test, the insulin response test can be a helpful tool to evaluate metabolic health and blood sugar regulation.

This test is similar to an OGTT (oral glucose tolerance test) and includes testing insulin at all intervals. The most common way of administering the OGTT with insulin response is first to collect a fasting sample and then samples at sixty minutes, ninety minutes, and 120 minutes following a seventy-five-gram glucose load (glucose syrup).

Understanding the insulin response can help determine the progression of diabetes or pre-diabetes and evaluate beta-cell dysfunction.

Fasting insulin: 2.5–6.0 uIU/mL

1–2 hour insulin: <30 uIU/mL

C-Peptide of Insulin

The c-peptide test is an important test to evaluate internal (endogenous) production of insulin, especially if you are using insulin therapy. The c-peptide is produced by the beta cells of the pancreas at the same rate as insulin. It's released when pro-insulin is divided and the insulin hormone is activated.

C-peptide has also been shown to have protective benefits against damage to brain cells and blood vessel walls by elevated glucose. When c-peptide levels are normal or high, it indicates functioning beta cells and can rule out beta-cell dysfunction.

C-peptide:

optimal 1.0–2.0 ng/mL

low <1.0 ng/mL

moderately high 2.1–4.0 ng/mL

high > 4.0 ng/mL

High-Sensitivity CRP

C-reactive protein is a protein component released by the liver in response to inflammation. It's been tested for many years to reveal infection after surgery or in other circumstances.

The high-sensitivity marker is used to evaluate the cardiovascular risk associated with inflammation. Additionally, studies have shown that elevated CRP indicates a higher risk of diabetes, hypertension, cancer, and dementia.

hsCRP:

normal <1.0 mg/L

moderate 1.0–3.0 mg/L

high >3.0 mg/L

Magnesium (Serum or RBC)

Only 25 percent of Americans consume the U.S. RDA of magnesium, and that level is considered by many health experts to be too low. Less than 1 percent of body magnesium is in the blood, and the serum magnesium level may not represent sufficiency.

Magnesium serum: 2.0–2.5 mg/dL

Magnesium RBC: 4.0–6.4 mg/dL

Vitamin B12

Vitamin B12 is an essential nutrient for nerve and blood cell health. It's also important for DNA replication. Therefore, insufficiency can lead to reduced cell replication and cause fatigue, weakness, irritability, and nerve problems.

It's also important to note that the drug metformin is known to deplete vitamin B12 levels.

Vitamin B12 serum: 400–1,000 pg/mL

If you are suspicious of vitamin B12 deficiency, it may be valuable to test homocysteine levels and methylmalonic acid (MMA).

Homocysteine is a metabolite released as a byproduct of protein metabolism that causes an inflammatory response. High homocysteine levels are a reliable risk indicator for heart disease and dementia. The body uses folate with B6 and B12 to convert homocysteine into other more useful compounds.

MMA is a metabolite that is elevated in 98 percent of people with B12 deficiency.

Homocysteine: <10 umol/L

MMA: 0.07–0.27 umol/L

Vitamin D

The standard vitamin D test is the 25-hydroxy immunoassay and is widely regarded as the most practical test. Another marker used less often is 1,25-dihidroxy vitamin D. This measures the bioactive form of vitamin D and can be useful in identifying the source of chronic vitamin D deficiency.

Low levels of vitamin D have been shown to have a strong correlation with the prevalence of diabetes through numerous studies. Recent research has demonstrated vitamin D receptors on the surfaces of pancreatic beta cells, which has opened a new avenue of investigation for the mechanism of vitamin D related to insulin function.

25-hydroxy vitamin D: 40–70 ng/dL

1,25-dihydroxy vitamin D: 18–72 pg/dL

Thyroid Testing

Thyroid hormone levels and activity are among the most critical and under-addressed factors in blood sugar health.

There are direct correlations reported in the research between low thyroid levels and insulin resistance, leading to high blood sugar and diabetes. The standard guidelines recommend TSH testing, but research and clinical experience have indicated inadequacy in that recommendation. It's useful to test thyroid hormones (T4, T3) directly to develop a complete understanding of thyroid physiology.

TSH: 1.0–2.0 mIU/mL

Thyroxine (T4): 7.0–10 ug/dL

Tri-iodothyronine (T3): 100–180 ng/dL

Free T4: 0.9–1.8 ng/dL

Free T3: 300–450 pg/dL, also reported as 3.0–4.5 pg/dL

There are circumstances where it's essential to evaluate autoimmune thyroid disease (Hashimoto's thyroiditis) using thyroid antibody testing. Elevations in reverse T3 often accompany leptin and insulin resistance. Elevated cortisol levels can have this same effect.

TPO antibody : <20 IU/mL

Thyroglobulin antibody: <8.0 IU/mL

THE MISSING TEST

Sharon came to my office frustrated with her doctor and her lack of results. She told me that she had had "every test available" and handed me a stack of papers dating back almost ten years. There were years of standard blood tests, adrenal tests, food sensitivity panels, even hair tests for heavy metal toxicity. None of the tests could make sense of her condition.

When she started with my program, Sharon was about sixty pounds overweight (clinically obese), and her blood sugar and hemoglobin A1c were in the pre-diabetic range. Her doctor told her that she was insulin resistant but had never tested her insulin level.

We sent her for some simple tests, like the ones described in this chapter, and found some stunning results. Her fasting insulin level was 48.2 (normal is <6.0). Her triglyceride levels were 186 (optimal is <70), and her hsCRP was 3.4 (optimal is <0.8). She was extremely insulin resistant, was likely dealing with fatty liver disease, and was on the road to becoming diabetic.

Sharon started the ProFAST diet and, within weeks, noticed a remarkable difference. The swelling in her wrists and ankles was gone. Her sugar and carbohydrate cravings vanished. Her energy soared, and the weight started melting off. After ten weeks, she had lost over thirty pounds, and her blood sugar was less than ninety most mornings (it had been averaging around 115–120).

When we repeated her lab tests, her physician couldn't believe the results. Not only had she lost weight and reversed her metabolic disease, but her triglycerides also dropped to ninety-two, her hsCRP was 1.4, and her fasting insulin level was down to twelve. Her health was not perfect, but she had achieved significant changes. The best part was how Sharon felt. She told me that we saved her life and marriage and that she felt like a new person. She was proud and excited about her new body, the health changes she had made, and what she was able to accomplish.

Understanding what's going on inside the body can be the motivating factor that can fuel your commitment to change. In most cases, blood glucose, basic lipids, and hemoglobin A1c, while important, are not enough to get the full picture. Evaluating insulin levels, liver enzymes, and other metabolic health markers can help determine the cause of high blood sugar, type-2 diabetes, and weight gain. It also enables you and your physician to track progress to achieve the best results.

CHAPTER 11

SUPPLEMENTING THE PROFAST DIET

Over the past hundred years, there have been countless "fad diets" propagated. They have ranged from the mundane and innocent, like the the Zone Diet, to the bizarre and dangerous, like the tapeworm diet, the cigarette diet, and the incredible cotton ball diet, which encouraged people to eat cotton balls to reduce hunger.[199] In the 1930s, a particularly dangerous trend toward liquid diets started to emerge. It began with Dr. Stoll's Aid and continued with the Master Cleanse and the cabbage soup diet, eventually leading to SlimFast and other more modern concoctions.[200]

One of these liquid-only diets proved to be particularly dangerous. It was called the "Last Chance Diet," created by osteopath Robert Linn.[201] While on this diet, the only thing people were allowed to consume was Dr. Linn's specially formulated collagen drink mix. This product was an artificially sweetened, low-quality protein drink made from slaughterhouse leftover products and chemical additives.

After close evaluation, it was determined that the drink mix was low in vitamins, minerals, electrolytes, and protein. Participants would spend four to six months living only on this liquid concoction, and unfortunately, dozens of people died. Upon examination, they found that most of these people had shrunken their heart muscle and suffered from cardiac problems.[202]

When Drs. Blackburn and Bistrian created the protein-sparing modified fast in the early 1970s, their objective was to help their patients maintain lean body mass while reducing excess fat. In their original papers, they advised that the program be done using whole foods and supplemented with vitamins, minerals, and electrolytes.[203] Later adaptations to the program have evolved to include essential fatty acid supplementation as well.[204]

We can learn from past medical mistakes, like the Last Chance Diet, that the body thrives on whole, real foods, and that if we're going to restrict energy to increase fat loss, we need to focus on optimizing micronutrients.

VITAL SUPPLEMENTS

The ProFAST diet is structured to maximize nutrient density while minimizing energy-dense foods. Fibrous vegetables such as spinach, broccoli, cauliflower, and berries are loaded with micronutrients. High-quality proteins—organic eggs, grass-fed beef, wild-caught fish, seafood, and pasture-raised chicken and turkey—are highly nutrient rich, containing essential vitamins, minerals, carotenoids, fatty acids, and other compounds.

In addition to the nutrient dense foods on the ProFAST diet, we recommend supplementing the diet with a few key products. These will ensure that you have adequate micronutrients to optimize health, balance your minerals and electrolytes, and recharge the essential fatty acid pool for your cells.

HIGH-QUALITY MULTIVITAMIN, MINERAL, AND PHYTONUTRIENT BLEND

Multivitamins are the most common and popular supplement sold in the world. Unfortunately, most products are ineffective and poorly made. There are thirteen essential vitamins and at least sixteen essential minerals without which humans cannot live. While most multivitamin formulas contain these essential vitamins and minerals, they come in various forms, many of which are poorly absorbed and virtually useless. There are also reports of misrepresentation of what is actually in the products.

Although many studies have shown that using multivitamin formulas offers little benefit to those already eating a healthy diet, there are some instances in which a high-quality formula can be helpful or even essential. Because the ProFAST diet is an energy-restricted eating plan, supplementation is highly recommended.

When choosing the right multivitamin, mineral, and nutrient formula, we recommend finding a professional product that uses only high-quality ingredients from reputable sources. Many blends follow the minimal RDA recommendations, where there is just enough of a nutrient to prevent deficiency disease. While this may help, it's not enough to ensure optimal health and vitality.

Australian researcher Dr. Michael Fenech has proposed that

RDA levels should be reexamined and revised to support current research around genomic stability, or healthy DNA replication in the cell.[205] These levels are higher in specific vitamins, like B12 and folate. Certain nutrients are especially critical for fat burning and blood sugar health, such as magnesium, chromium, vitamin D, vitamin K, and many B vitamins.

In addition to vitamins and minerals, there are also phytonutrients, which have tremendous health benefits to consider including in your multi.

Carotenoids like lutein and lycopene can protect cells from oxidative stress, improve brain function, and prevent particular health problems associated with high blood sugar.[206]

Muscadine grape extract and wild blueberry complex have potent antioxidant compounds that reduce inflammation, protect cells and organs such as the liver and cardiovascular system, inhibit AGEs (advanced glycation end products from high blood sugar), improve vision, and increase fat burning.[207]

Broccoli extract contains powerful glucosinolates, which improve detoxification and gut health.[208] Citrus bioflavonoids contain hesperidin, a compound found to reduce inflammation, relax blood vessels protecting the heart, support neurological function, and improve insulin sensitivity.[209]

Combining these powerful phytonutrients with the right doses of essential vitamins and minerals from high-quality sources will provide your body with the necessary micronutrients to thrive on the ProFAST diet.

ELECTROLYTES

Electrolytes are electrically charged minerals essential in many functions of the body, including muscle contraction, hydration, regulation of pH levels, and proper nerve function. Minerals exist in various states inside the body and are used for thousands of different reactions. Electrolytic minerals are dissolved in fluid and carry a positive or negative charge. This state allows them to move across cell membranes and throughout the body, pushing an electrical charge.

Electrolyte imbalances can have negative health consequences, leading to fatigue, confusion, headaches, muscle weakness or cramping, and irregular heartbeat, and in some cases, they may even be fatal. Typically, electrolyte imbalances are caused by dehydration, diuretics, blood sugar medications like SGLT2 inhibitors, diarrhea or vomiting, kidney disease, and excessive sweating.

Energy-restricted diets and diets known to stimulate ketone production can also cause a loss of electrolytes. One of the benefits of the ProFAST diet is that insulin levels will fall, which allows the body to burn fat more effectively. When insulin levels are low, the kidneys will excrete more sodium and water, which may disrupt other electrolyte levels in the body, such as potassium.

Many people, especially when transitioning from a moderate- or high-carbohydrate diet, experience something called the "low-carb flu" or "keto flu." When eating a large number of carbohydrates, the liver's and muscles' glycogen stores are filled, and there is fluid retention due to high circulating insulin levels. When insulin drops and liver glycogen is depleted, the body releases water, leading to mild dehydration and loss of electrolytes. Replacing the water and electrolytes has been shown to eliminate the symptoms associated with this phenomenon.

There are many food sources of these essential minerals on the ProFAST diet, including mushrooms, leafy green vegetables, Brussels sprouts, broccoli, salmon, flounder, artichoke, and beef. Sodium recommendations for those on an energy-restricted ketogenic diet are about 3–7 grams per day, and potassium is about 3.0–4.7 grams per day.

Many people find it helpful to add a good-quality salt, such as Redmond's Real Salt or Celtic sea salt to their food. It's also essential to add a supplemental electrolyte product while on the ProFAST diet.

When selecting an effective electrolyte product, we recommend choosing a professional product using purified ionic trace minerals from natural sources such as seawater. The product should contain a balance of the most critical electrolytes, including sodium, potassium, magnesium, zinc, chloride, and sulfate in an isosmotic solution so that it doesn't cause depletion of water or other ions.[210]

ESSENTIAL FATTY ACIDS

While there are no essential carbohydrates, there are essential vitamins, minerals, amino acids (protein), and fatty acids. Restricting energy in the form of carbohydrates and fat in the diet will upregulate fatty acid oxidation or fat burning in the cells and lead to significant fat loss. This increased fat utilization is one of the goals of the ProFAST diet. It's also crucial to optimize nutrient density, including essential fatty acids.

The essential fatty acids are essential because humans need

them to survive and cannot synthesize them internally. They include linoleic acid (an omega-6 polyunsaturated fat) and alpha-linolenic acid (an omega-3 polyunsaturated fat).

These fatty acids are critical structural components of cell membranes and are important precursors for other fatty acids. Linoleic acid is prevalent in most foods, including meats, eggs, freshwater fish, soy, and many vegetables. Alpha-linolenic acid is more difficult to obtain on an energy-restricted diet. Therefore, we recommend supplementing a good-quality fish oil containing ALA and preformed DHA and EPA.

The long-chain omega-3 fatty acids DHA and EPA can be synthesized by the body from ALA. Still, it's an energy-dependent process that is variable based on the availability of synthesizing enzymes and individual genetic variations. It's generally considered preferable to supply these valuable fatty acids directly through diet or supplementation.

DHA (docosahexaenoic acid) is vital for the brain and eyes and has been shown to improve cardiovascular health, reduce lipids, help with ADHD, speed muscle recovery, and fight inflammation.[211]

EPA (eicosapentaenoic acid) lowers triglycerides and LDL cholesterol, improves blood pressure, prevents blood clotting, reduces arterial plaquing, can prevent some forms of cancer, and helps to squelch systemic inflammation.[212]

When selecting the right fish oil product, quality is paramount. As with other supplements, we recommend choosing a professional brand with the highest quality standards. Omega-3 polyunsaturated fats are prone to oxidation, so it's wise to store the product carefully. Oxidation is facilitated by heat, light, and air, so it's best to store it in a dark cabinet or the refrigerator. Aim for at least 1,000 mg per day of combined DHA and EPA, and consider using 2–4 grams of fish oil per day.

OTHER SUPPLEMENTS

There are many other supplements that can be considered for certain situations, some of which are described here. It's important to discuss your specific supplement plan with a qualified health practitioner to safely optimize your nutritional strategy.

SUPPLEMENTAL FIBER

Many people find supplemental fiber helps with bowel patterns and provides additional satiety. The American Diabetes Association recommends that people get twenty-five to fifty grams of dietary fiber per day. Soluble and insoluble fiber improves the gut microbiome health, gut motility, glycemic response, and levels of cholesterol and triglycerides and provides more satiety or feelings of fullness.

The ProFAST diet includes high-fiber vegetables such as broccoli, Brussels sprouts, spinach, collards, chard, asparagus, kale, and cauliflower.

There are many different types of fiber, and instead of using only one fiber type, we recommend choosing a product with a variety of fiber types. These should be non-grain fibers, free of gluten, lectins, and phytates, and can include inulin, CreaFibe cellulose, carrot fiber, citrus fiber, apple pectin, flax, and glucomannan.

MAGNESIUM

Additional magnesium can help with sleep, relaxation, energy levels, headaches, exercise performance, feelings of depression, blood sugar, and muscle spasms.[213] In the form of magnesium citrate, it also draws water into the bowels, acting as an osmotic laxative and increasing bowel motility.[214]

If you have loose stools or experience diarrhea, use a chelated form of magnesium, such as magnesium malate, gluconate, or glycinate. These forms are more quickly absorbed through the gut and typically do not stimulate the bowels.

VITAMIN D

Extra vitamin D can improve immune function, blood sugar health, and bone health and reduce feelings of depression.[215] Studies have shown that vitamin D supplementation can protect against cardiovascular disease and improve weight loss, helping to reduce appetite.[216]

Vitamin D is produced in our skin cells from cholesterol when our skin is exposed to direct sunlight and can be found in many of the foods on the ProFAST diet, including salmon, eggs, shrimp, and yogurt.

However, recent studies indicate that around 42 percent of the U.S. population is deficient in vitamin D, which has been linked to obesity and type-2 diabetes. Therefore, vitamin D supplementation is widely recommended.

When choosing the right vitamin D product, it's best to use the most bioavailable form, vitamin D3. Although the RDA is just 800 IU per day, most of my clients find that they need 2,000–5,000 IU per day to maintain sufficient blood levels.

SUPERFOOD POWDER

One of the goals of the ProFAST diet is to strive for the highest nutrient density possible. This result is achieved by eating high-quality protein sources and fibrous vegetables. For people who want to boost their nutrient consumption, there is nothing better than using a superfood powder.

This product is a combination of dehydrated fruit and vegetable powders that contains high levels of micronutrients with very little energy from carbohydrates or fat. For example, one typical serving might contain the equivalent micronutrient content of fifteen servings of fruits and vegetables with only two grams of fat and net carbohydrates.

These products provide potent antioxidant benefits, enhance immune function, provide alkalizing minerals, support liver health and detoxification, and provide digestive enzymes, probiotics, and healthy fiber.

As recommended with other products, it's good to choose a professional product blend that uses trustworthy ingredients and is third-party inspected to ensure accuracy and quality.

Most other nutrient-based supplements can be safely consumed while on the ProFAST diet. I generally recommend suspending botanical agents, such as high-dose cinnamon, berberine, and other herbs, as these may artificially lower blood sugar, leading to hypoglycemia, or have other unintended consequences.

A SIMPLE SOLUTION

I talked to Marjorie several times per week for over a month, trying to help her solve her most recent problems. She was one of my best clients. When Marjorie started her journey toward beating diabetes, her blood sugar was averaging just below 200 mg/dl, and she had gained about thirty pounds. She was eager to make changes and get results.

After implementing some dietary changes, Marjorie almost immediately started to lose weight, and her blood sugar dropped below 100 into a healthy range. Unfortunately, she had other problems. She wasn't sleeping very well, and her energy was terrible. She didn't feel very well.

Over the next few months, we worked on her sleep routine, and she saw significant improvements. But she still didn't feel great. Finally, while Marjorie was telling me how much water she was drinking (twice the average of most of my clients), I thought her electrolytes might be out of balance.

Marjorie began adding real salt to her foods and water and included an electrolyte product with her daily routine. It was almost like magic. Within days, her energy started climbing, her sleep improved, she could start exercising again, and she felt like a new person.

Often, the answer is not the most complicated solution but something simple and straightforward. It's about finding the right combination to open the lock that allows the body to function the way it was designed to work.

The ProFAST diet is an energy-restricted eating plan and should be supplemented with the right combination of vitamins, minerals, phytonutrients, fatty acids, and electrolytes. This approach can help prevent deficiencies, protect your health, and enhance your results and experience.

CHAPTER 12

ODDS AND ENDS

From ancient Indian texts, there's a story about a group of blind men. These men had heard rumors of a new animal that had come into town. It was called an elephant. They sought out the animal in order to understand it.

Once they were brought to the animal, they each began to touch it and describe what they felt. The first man said, "It feels like a snake," as he ran his hands along the trunk.

The next said, "It feels more like a tree," as he placed his hand on the elephant's leg.

A third said, "It's more like a rope than a snake" as he held the animal's tail.

And the fourth man said, "It feels like a solid wall to me," as he laid his hands on the elephant's side.

After the men shared their experience, they realized that they only saw the animal from their limited perspective and there was much more to discover once they were open to learning more.

Each person who follows the ProFAST diet will have a unique experience and will have their perspective. Understanding the plan more fully will help you have a more profound experience and increase the likelihood of significant results.

FREQUENTLY ASKED QUESTIONS

These questions were compiled from my experience working with hundreds of clients engaging in the ProFAST diet, and assimilating the answers will help you develop a deeper understanding of the program and allow you to get through most of the challenges and obstacles that you may encounter.

WHAT ARE TYPICAL RESULTS OF THE PROFAST DIET?

As you might imagine, there is no such thing as a "typical result." Everyone is different and, therefore, will achieve different results using the ProFAST diet. The good news is that based on my twenty years of experience supervising this program with thousands of patients and clients, everyone will achieve some level of positive results.

Studies on the protein-sparing modified fast have demonstrated significant weight loss and improvements in blood sugar and HbA1c. One study done at the Cleveland Clinic showed an average weight loss of twenty-five pounds and a 10 percent reduction in body weight.[217] Another published in the *American Journal of Clinical Nutrition* found that in six weeks, participants lost an average of thirty-two pounds of body fat with no loss of lean muscle mass.[218]

Specific results will depend on your starting point, considering your weight, body fat and glycemic control, amount of insulin resistance, and insulin levels. It's also determined by the level of intensity that you choose, your compliance with the program, and other factors such as thyroid function, sleep quality, and stress.

Be confident that you will achieve positive results, and commit to following through with the program, regardless of the day-to-day changes you're seeing. It's better to make a full evaluation at the end of the program than micro-assess your daily progress.

IS THE PROFAST DIET SAFE?

This program is adapted from the protein-sparing modified fast, which has been studied extensively in clinical trials. It's been safely used by thousands of people, including overweight men and women, adolescents (in clinical trials), and elite bodybuilders aiming to cut fat and become ultra-lean.

One study concluded that the protein-sparing modified fast could be safely and effectively used in an outpatient environment for rapid weight loss.[219]

As with any energy-restricted eating plan, it's good to inform your doctor before starting and to have medical supervision throughout the program. For example, at the Cleveland Clinic, patients using a PSMF meet with a dietitian regularly during the program and with a nurse practitioner every six to eight weeks to monitor labs and address symptoms.[220]

Because the ProFAST diet is less restrictive and includes three intensity levels based on individual goals, body fatness, and situation, it is considered very safe.

For a description of common symptoms during the ProFAST diet, see the question below.

This program should not be used by children, pregnant or nursing women, and people with advanced cancer or type-1 diabetes or who are underweight. Further, those with a history of gallstones, ketoacidosis, dehydration, chronic kidney disease, untreated hypo-thyroidism, eating disorders, or gout should use extreme caution with the program and must be closely medically supervised.

WHAT ARE THE MOST COMMON SYMPTOMS WHILE ON THE PROFAST DIET?

If you've ever used an energy-restricted diet, you know that there's a possibility of symptoms at various stages of the program. Fortunately, most of these can be solved and overcome with a few simple strategies. The most common symptoms during the ProFAST diet include headache, constipation, dehydration, fatigue, cold intolerance, halitosis, dry skin, and lightheadedness.

The majority of these symptoms are solved with the recommended supplements, including 1,000 mg of a high DHA and EPA fish oil; a specially designed, high-quality multivitamin, multi-mineral supplement; and an electrolyte formula. Additionally, many people find that supplemental fiber and extra magnesium may help prevent infrequent stools.

Eating more protein can lead to dehydration and mineral loss, so in addition to the recommended supplements, it's essential to stay well hydrated on the ProFAST diet. We recommend consuming at least one ounce of water per half pound of body weight.

HOW SHOULD I DETERMINE THE PATH OF INTENSITY TO FOLLOW DURING THE ENGAGEMENT PHASE?

There are certain parts of the ProFAST diet, such as protein recommendations related to body requirements, that are based on optimal body weight and fat mass. However, the other macronutrients, fat, and carbohydrate consumption are based more on your individual goals and how quickly and aggressively you want to lose weight (as well as your body fat percentage).

As described in Chapter 8, there are three paths of varying intensity that you can choose for yourself based on your starting point and your goals:

- Level 1: Moderate. The moderate plan is for people who are looking for significant changes in body fat loss and blood sugar reduction at a steady pace. This path is typically for men with an estimated body fat percentage of greater than 15 percent and women with an estimated body fat percentage of greater than 20 percent.
- Level 2: Accelerated. The accelerated plan is for people who are looking for more serious changes in body fatness and need to lower blood sugar levels and reduce insulin resistance significantly. This path is typically for men with an estimated body fat percentage of greater than 20 percent and women with an estimated body fat percentage of greater than 25 percent.
- Level 3: Aggressive. The intensive plan is for people who are looking for major changes in body fat, blood sugar levels, and insulin sensitivity and those who want to reverse prediabetes or type-2 diabetes while minimizing the need for diabetes medications. This path is typically for men with an estimated body fat percentage of greater than 25 percent and women with an estimated body fat percentage of greater than 30 percent.

Even if you meet the requirements and description for Level 3, it doesn't mean that you must start there. Some people start with the moderate or accelerated plan, increasing the intensity once they feel comfortable with the program. Likewise, it's acceptable to reduce intensity level based on your feelings, symptoms, negative lab findings, or physician's advice.

CAN I DO THE PROGRAM FOR A SHORTER OR LONGER AMOUNT OF TIME?

It's highly recommended that you follow the ProFAST diet as described in this book for optimal results. Quitting the program early or skipping the transition phase often leads to weight gain and elevated blood sugar levels back to the original starting point or sometimes worse.

Studies on the protein-sparing modified fast have been performed for six months successfully. However, results will steadily decrease throughout that time, yielding diminishing returns, and there is a much higher chance of relapse and regain during extended programs.

In my experience over twenty years working with thousands of patients and clients on the ProFAST diet, the optimal engagement period is six to eight weeks, followed by four weeks of transition to reset homeostatic control through the hypothalamus.

If you need to stop the program due to serious symptoms, negative lab findings, or at your physician's request, then you can do so safely by increasing your carbohydrate and fat consumption to maintenance levels right away. Then, work with your doctor to optimize macronutrients to improve your long-term health outcomes.

CAN I DO THE PROFAST DIET AS A VEGETARIAN OR VEGAN OR USING A PLANT-BASED DIET?

Yes! While it's typically easier to follow the ProFAST diet while incorporating animal protein, there are various protein options for those following a vegetarian, vegan, or plant-based diet.

The majority of the menu, by volume, consists of some low-glycemic fruit and an abundance of fibrous vegetables. Plant-based protein sources include whole soy (including tofu), nutritional yeast, cottage cheese, Greek yogurt, peanut powder, and high-quality plant-based protein powder.

If you are a vegan, be sure to include the multivitamin and electrolyte formula and substitute an algae-based omega-3 product for fish oil.

CAN I CHEW GUM, HAVE BREATH MINTS, OR USE FLAVORED WATER DURING THE PROFAST DIET?

Most people find that chewing gum while on an energy-restricted eating plan will make them hungrier and stimulate sugar cravings. Additionally, many artificial sweeteners in commercially produced chewing gum have been shown to increase appetite and harm the gut microbiome, leading to weight gain and insulin resistance.[221] Therefore, we recommend avoiding chewing gum if possible.

Likewise, most breath mints are sweetened using artificial sweeteners and should be avoided. There are gum and mint products sweetened with low-calorie, natural sweeteners that may be acceptable in limited quantities. Mints and gum that contains xylitol should be avoided due to the net carbohydrates and calories associated with this sugar alcohol.

Instead of gum or breath mints, we recommend using a natural peppermint breath spray made with peppermint essential oil to combat adverse breath symptoms.

Flavored drops for water can be used as long as they contain the acceptable sweeteners, such as stevia, erythritol, or monk fruit extract. We've found that some people tend to drink more water when using these drops, which can help with hydration on the ProFAST diet.

SHOULD I CONTINUE MY MEDICATIONS OR SUPPLEMENTS WHILE ON THE PROFAST DIET?

Most medications and supplements can be continued on the ProFAST diet, with a few precautions. If you are using insulin or oral diabetes medications that cause insulin release, such as sulfonylureas, meglitinides, or other secretagogues, it's helpful to discuss the eating plan and medication management with your physician. Also, blood pressure often drops during the ProFAST diet, so hypertensive medications should be monitored closely.

If you are taking potent blood sugar-lowering supplements, such as Berberine, closely monitor your blood sugar, especially as it approaches the normal range. It might be best to reduce or discontinue these supplements as the plan progresses. Nutrient-based supplements, such as probiotics and vitamin D, can be continued as recommended by your qualified healthcare practitioner.

Additionally, it's essential to take the recommended supplements, including a high-quality multivitamin, multi-mineral formula, fish oil, and electrolytes.

As with any new eating plan or exercise program, it's recommended to discuss the details with your physician, including medication management, to help you use the most effective strategy to stay safe and get results.

SHOULD I EXERCISE WHILE DOING THE PROFAST DIET?

Exercise and physical activity are part of a healthy lifestyle and may be continued during the ProFAST diet, with a few guidelines. Slow, fat-burning, aerobic cardiovascular exercise, such as walking, biking, and swimming, are excellent ways to increase energy expenditure, improve cardiometabolic fitness, and increase fat oxidation.

I recommend thirty to sixty minutes of aerobic physical activity per day, whenever possible. Short-duration resistance training, such as bodyweight exercise, can also stimulate lean muscle preservation and growth and deplete muscle glycogen to improve insulin sensitivity. You can also consider adding "micro-workouts," which are described earlier in this book.

High-intensity cardiovascular or resistance exercise or prolonged high-exertion physical activity should be avoided during the ProFAST diet. This type of training puts additional stress on the adrenal glands and liver to produce glucose and stimulate the appetite.

WHAT SUPPLEMENTS SHOULD I TAKE OR NOT TAKE DURING THE PROFAST DIET?

As described in the book and the answers to other questions listed here, we recommend three essential supplements during the ProFAST diet. According to research by Drs. Blackburn and Bistrian, creators of the original protein-sparing modified fast, a high-quality multivitamin, multi-mineral formula, and electrolyte blend should be used during this program.

We've created a specific formula called Super Multi, which contains a broad spectrum of essential nutrients in their optimal forms and vital phytochemicals such as lutein, quercetin, citrus bioflavonoids, resveratrol, and a variety of other superfood antioxidants and plant compounds.

Additionally, we've created an electrolyte product called Electro Balance, which contains a blend of ionic trace minerals such as magnesium, zinc, chloride, sodium, and potassium in the most easily absorbed and usable forms.

Lastly, we recommend a high-quality fish oil product with concentrated DHA and EPA fatty acids to ensure the consumption of essential fatty acids. Use a product that contains at least 1,000 mg of combined EPA and DHA per serving, and take one to two servings per day.

Other supplements may be helpful, including additional magnesium, fiber, probiotics, and fat-soluble vitamins such as vitamins A, D, E, and K.

WHAT SHOULD I DO IF I CANNOT GET LABS DONE?

In most cases, lab tests are not essential to begin the ProFAST diet but can help evaluate progress. If you have kidney disease or advanced liver disease or you take medications known to affect electrolyte balance, it's highly recommended to have a full lab evaluation before beginning the program.

One research paper describing a similar dietary approach recommended having several tests before starting the program, including a CBC; comprehensive metabolic panel with electrolytes, liver enzymes, and kidney tests; lipid profile; thyroid testing; glucose; HbA1c; and uric acid.[222]

For most people, lab testing is not required, but it's important to discuss this with your physician before starting the ProFAST diet.

WHAT SHOULD I DO IF I CAN'T GET MY DOCTOR ON BOARD WITH THE PROGRAM?

Many physicians are hesitant to recommend an energy-restricted eating plan, even though there is ample evidence published in the literature showing that it's highly effective for weight loss, blood sugar control, reduction of HbA1c, lipid metabolism, and long-term cardiovascular health.[223]

I recommend visiting profastdiet.com to research and download the papers supporting the protein-sparing modified fast and VLCDs for managing type-2 diabetes, obesity, and blood sugar. Print these studies and share them with your physician. Helping your doctor understand the evidence base supporting this program will likely encourage them to consider the option.

If you feel strongly about using the ProFAST diet, share your commitment with your physician, and let them know that you'd like them to monitor you through the process to ensure your safety. We do not recommend starting the ProFAST diet without your doctor's knowledge or without having medical supervision.

WHAT IS THE BEST WAY TO HANDLE HUNGER OR FOOD CRAVINGS DURING THE ENGAGEMENT PHASE?

The first thing to understand here is that there are two types of hunger. The first type of hunger is emotional. It's not real physiological hunger but rather a deep desire to eat something. People want to eat for many reasons. Some eat because they are bored; others because they are stressed, and others to enjoy the taste of food. None of these reasons have anything to do with actual hunger.

Physiological hunger emanates from a need for protein, energy, and micronutrients. All of these factors can drive real hunger, but most often, it's the need for micronutrients and protein. Most people interested in following the ProFAST diet have plenty of stored energy, so the requirement for external energy is minimal.

Many people experience intense food cravings for snacks, sweets, and energy-rich foods (fat and carbohydrate). While these types of feelings are difficult to overcome, it's best not to indulge in bad behavior for a quick but fleeting sense of gratification. The long-term benefits of breaking these cravings will be well worth the effort.

When you're feeling a desire to eat extra food in the program, it's important to ask yourself if you are truly hungry. Is this feeling based on mental or emotional stress or boredom? Is it an escape from something you're dealing with in life? Do you miss the taste of a particular food or the act of eating something that you like?

If so, it's best not to indulge in this type of pathological eating strategy. Instead, go for a walk, take a shower, call a friend, or drink some hot tea. The feeling will typically fade within fifteen to twenty minutes or become less powerful.

If you determine that you are genuinely physiologically hungry, the first solution is to drink sixteen ounces of water. Then, eat a large salad in a giant bowl filled with leafy greens, cucumbers, mushrooms, and other fibrous vegetables. If you are still physiologically hungry, eat one to two ounces of additional lean protein, such as a hard-boiled egg or two (one yolk only).

After eating a nutrient-rich salad and extra protein, if you still feel hungry, you know it's emotional hunger, not physiological.

WHAT SHOULD I DO IF I EXPERIENCE IRRITABILITY, FATIGUE, OR BRAIN FOG?

Probably the most common symptom people will experience during the ProFAST diet is a feeling of fatigue. If this happens early in the engagement phase, it is typically related to the shift in fuel utilization from external energy sources (carbs and fat in food) to internal sources (stored body fat).

The process of mitochondrial adaptation to upregulate fat burning can take up to four weeks. During this time, it's possible to experience some fatigue, lightheadedness, hunger, and irritability. The solution is to rest when necessary, continue to stay the course, and allow your body to start burning more fat and producing more ketones, which are an alternative energy source the body uses during a fasted or low-energy state.

Another potential source of fatigue is electrolyte imbalance. Make sure that you are using a quality electrolyte product, and consider increasing the number of electrolytes that you take each day. For example, you may want to escalate from one serving per day to two. Likewise, hydration is essential. If you feel tired, increase your water intake by sixteen ounces per day (do not exceed one ounce per pound of body weight).

Fatigue may also come from the detoxification associated with energy-restricted eating plans. When you follow an energy-restricted program, your body increases autophagy and upregulates phase-one detoxification in the liver, increasing circulating toxins and creating a feeling of fatigue, headache, and irritability.

In this case, we recommend supplementing a detoxification support product and adding a binder such as activated charcoal or fiber. See the resources section for more information.

If you feel fatigued later in the engagement phase, after week four, it could be related to the downregulation of thyroid hormone levels if the fatigue is accompanied by cold intolerance, hair loss, or constipation. In this case, I recommend adding some additional carbohydrates (10–20 grams) to your daily plan, typically with the dinner meal, as healthy starch.

Alternatively, you can do a "refeed day," which is explained earlier in this book. The downregulation of thyroid hormone during fasting or an energy-restricted eating plan is temporary and will self-correct once you move into the transition phase and maintenance.

I'VE BEEN FEELING SLIGHTLY CONSTIPATED ON THE PROFAST DIET. WHAT IS THE BEST WAY TO HANDLE THIS?

First, let's define constipation. Constipation is considered infrequent or incomplete bowel movements and less than three bowel movements per week. It's entirely reasonable for bowel patterns to slow while fasting or on an energy-restricted diet, as there is much less volume moving through the digestive tract. Additionally, if you had been consuming grain or grain-based products, consider that these often contain lectins and insoluble fibers that irritate and stimulate the gut. On a grain-free diet, you rely on low-glycemic vegetables for the majority of your dietary fiber.

If your bowel movements feel hard or uncomfortable due to difficulty moving the bowels, you may want to consider adding more soluble fiber through a high-quality fiber supplement. It's also important to make sure you are well hydrated by drinking at least half your body weight in water each day.

To increase bowel motility, you can try adding 300–400 mg of magnesium citrate in the evening. Many people have also found relief from high-dose probiotics. Consider adding a high-quality professional probiotic product and consuming 100 billion CFUs per day to support gut motility.

I do not generally recommend using laxatives or stool softeners. However, if you are medically constipated and have not had a bowel movement in more than three days, you may consider using a natural senna leaf tea to stimulate the bowels. Note that this may cause abdominal cramping.

If constipation persists for more than one week, consider a "refeed day" with higher carbohydrates, as described earlier. Consult your physician if constipation continues, if you feel that you need medical attention, or if you develop severe abdominal pain.

I'M BORED WITH THE FOOD CHOICES ON THE PROFAST DIET. HOW CAN I MAKE THIS MORE INTERESTING?

As one of my clients said to me, "I can do this. It may be boring, but boring doesn't kill you." This statement reveals an interesting and critical perspective. Obesity, type-2 diabetes, pre-diabetes, insulin resistance, Alzheimer's disease, and cardiovascular problems will kill you. Simple, healthy, nutrient-dense food will not. It will likely save your life.

There is a shift that most of us need to make at one point or another away from using food as entertainment toward using food for nourishment. Once you make that shift, food is no longer boring or exciting. Food becomes more nourishing or less nourishing, more nutrient dense or less nutrient dense. That change in perspective will have profoundly positive effects on your health and life.

If you want to make the engagement phase of the ProFAST diet more enjoyable, there are dozens of delicious recipes in this book. Ultimately, we recommend finding a few meals that you enjoy and rotating those throughout the week. Typically, the simpler you make this plan, the more successful you'll be with the program. And remember, boring doesn't kill you.

WHAT HAPPENS IF I DON'T GET ENOUGH PROTEIN OR HAVE A HARD TIME EATING THE PROTEIN RECOMMENDATIONS ON THE PROFAST DIET?

The ProFAST diet is an adaptation of a dietary, medical intervention called the protein-sparing modified fast. The PSMF was created in the 1970s by renowned nutritional scientists and physicians Drs. Blackburn and Bistrian as a way to preserve lean body mass while losing significant amounts of fat mass. Research by these doctors and others has shown that consuming 1.5 grams of protein per kilogram of ideal body weight will protect muscle from breakdown during long-term energy restriction.[224]

Adequate protein consumption not only allows optimal nitrogen balance (muscle sparing) but also is highly satiating and helps you feel full and satisfied. According to the creators of the protein leverage hypothesis, Drs. Simpson and Raubenheimer, the human metabolism prioritizes protein, and we will eat until we get adequate protein.[225] Therefore, ensuring optimal protein consumption will prevent overeating and help to suppress appetite.

Make protein your priority. Focus on getting enough protein throughout the day, and fill the rest of your diet with leafy greens and other nutrient dense, low-glycemic vegetables.

MY WEIGHT OR BLOOD SUGAR HAS STALLED DURING THE ENGAGEMENT PHASE AND IS NOT COMING DOWN OR HAS GONE UP. HOW CAN I BREAK THROUGH THIS PLATEAU?

Almost everyone doing the ProFAST diet will hit a stall or a plateau of weight or blood sugar changes at some point during the program. It's an entirely normal part of the body's adaptation process and should not be interpreted as negative or discouraging.

Before we discuss how to overcome this state, let's first discuss what a "plateau" actually is and is not. We define a stall or plateau as four consecutive days with no significant net progress in weight loss. Weight may fluctuate from day to day but should be trending down throughout the program's engagement phase.

Blood sugar levels may plateau independent of weight loss and should be managed differently. If you have reached a point with no net progress in weight loss over four consecutive days, you can use the following strategies to break through that plateau.

First, evaluate yourself for compliance. Make sure you are closely tracking what and how much you are eating, and not overconsuming carbohydrates or fat energy. It's very easy to overeat if you are just "eyeballing" your meals rather than closely tracking your food intake.

Secondly, evaluate your physical activity. If you are overdoing resistance training, it can lead to muscle hypertrophy (swelling), causing an increase in glycogen storage and water retention in the muscles. This swelling is not a bad thing, but it will increase your weight and hide changes from fat loss.

Third, evaluate your bowel patterns. Often, weight loss appears to stall because you haven't moved your bowels and the intestinal tract is full. Follow the recommendations for alleviating constipation if this is an issue.

If you've evaluated these areas and still feel like you have reached a plateau with your weight, there are two modifications that you can use to overcome the plateau.

The first modification is called a superfood fiber fast (SF3) and is much closer to a full water fast. In addition to water and coffee, tea, or other non-caloric, unsweetened beverages, during the SF3 day, you'll consume six to eight servings of a superfood powder (greens powder) with an added serving of high-quality fiber.

The SF3 day starts upon waking and ends with the introduction of food the next day. You may also want to consider adding some magnesium citrate or a gentle laxative tea in the evening of the SF3 day.

The second modification is called PROMAD and involves one day with a time-restricted eating window of only one hour and eating one small ProFAST meal in the evening (OMAD).

For example, you would drink water, coffee, tea, or other non-caloric, unsweetened beverages throughout the day with no other food. Then, from six o'clock to seven o'clock in the evening (or whatever one-hour eating window is appropriate), you would consume one small ProFast meal with no more than four ounces of protein, minimal carbohydrates from leafy greens or low-glycemic vegetables, and no added fat.

Regardless of which strategy you try, the regular ProFAST Diet should be continued the next day. In the majority of cases, these strategies will help you break through a weight plateau. However, even if your weight does not change, it's essential to follow the regular ProFAST Diet for four to five days before attempting another modification.

Lastly, make sure you look at the big picture. If you've already lost considerable weight, it's possible that your body needs to take a few days to reset your homeostatic weight balance. There are various dynamics associated with weight, including hydration, electrolyte balance, bowel contents, muscle hypertrophy, liver and muscle glycogen storage, and fluid retention.

Be patient and give your body time to adjust. Most of the time, people move through short plateaus on the ProFAST diet without doing anything different. Consistency is often the key to long-term change.

A FEW WORDS ABOUT SUPPORT

One of the most critical determinants for success on the Pro-FAST diet is your support system. If you can recruit a friend, family member, or other acquaintance to do the program with you or agree to support you through the process, you'll find the plan much more rewarding and comfortable to follow.

If you need additional outside support, you are welcome to join the ProFast community by visiting our website at profastdiet. com or joining our Facebook group. There, we have encouraging discussions every day, where participants can post their questions and get support from each other and the moderators.

Whichever way you choose to set up your support system, I do not recommend trying to do this alone. Making changes to lose weight, improve blood sugar, and beat diabetes is challenging. Don't make it harder on yourself. Find a person, small local group, or global community like ours to help you stay encouraged, motivated, and on the right path toward successful change.

CONCLUSION

You've made it to the end of this book, probably feeling excited about the possibilities but a little anxious about getting started. You might be wondering, "Where do I begin?"

That's completely normal. I recommend starting by getting your plan organized and getting yourself prepared.

Seth Godin, the Stanford-trained entrepreneur and bestselling author has said, "The only thing worse than starting something and failing is not starting something." Don't expect yourself to be perfect or to figure everything out in advance. Just get started.

The ProFAST diet is designed to help you succeed with rapid fat loss, better blood sugar, less insulin resistance, more energy, increased metabolic health, and reversal of type-2 diabetes so that you can reduce or eliminate medication.

The program will help you feel satiated, have less sugar and carbohydrate cravings, protect lean body mass while encouraging fat loss, and give you more energy and a clearer mind.

In the beginning of the book, I discussed the truth about type-2 diabetes and metabolic health, including the problem with insulin and how high insulin levels lead to fat accumulation and high blood sugar.

Then, I described nutrient and energy density, the protein-to-energy ratio, and the importance of protein for increasing metabolic rate and protecting lean body mass, including muscle.

This was followed with the science of fasting, revealing the benefits of intermittent fasting and time-restricted eating, including the production of ketones, reduction in insulin, increase in autophagy, and rebuilding of healthy body tissue. Ketones, as I discussed next, fuel the muscles, brain, and heart, leading to reduced appetite, less muscle loss, and increased energy.

In the second half of the book, I went through the details of the ProFAST diet, outlining the step-by-step program to achieve your goals successfully. I discussed how to calculate your macronutrients, optimize your protein-to-energy ratio, the foods to eat and those to avoid, and how to incorporate physical activity in your plan.

I discussed how to transition to a long-term plan to maintain positive changes without losing momentum or progress. I went over lab testing and evaluation and the most important supplements to consider while on the ProFAST diet. Finally, I answered common questions that many people have before starting or while on the program.

Hopefully, this book has given you hope and created some excitement about what is possible for you if you're willing to put in the time and effort to get results.

In this book, you have all the tools and resources you need to succeed with the program. To help support you in the process, we've also created a website with tools, resources, additional recipes, a section for your physician, and links to relevant studies. If you want or need some extra guidance or help, visit the website at profastdiet.com.

My hope and desire are that after reading *The ProFAST Diet*, you are eager and excited to make the necessary changes and follow the program to reach your goals. This program has changed my life and the lives of hundreds of my patients and clients over the years. Maybe it can change yours as well.

RECIPES

SHRIMP DEVILED EGGS

Serves 2

Energy 127 kcal | Protein 17g | Fat 6g | Net Carbs 3g | P:E Ratio 2:1

Ingredients:

- 4 eggs (2 yolks only)
- 1 tsp tabasco
- 1/4 cup low-fat plain Greek yogurt (Two Good) (2.5 oz)
- 1 pinch herbal salt
- 8 large cooked and peeled shrimp
- Fresh dill

Instructions:

- Place the eggs in a pot and cover them with water. Place the pot over medium heat and bring to a light boil. Boil for 8–10 minutes to make sure the eggs are hard-boiled. Remove the eggs from the pot and place in an ice bath or cold water for a few minutes before peeling.

- Split the eggs in half and scoop out the yolks. You will only use half of the yolks. Place the egg whites on a plate. Mash the yolks with a fork and add tabasco, herbal salt, and low-fat plain Greek yogurt. Add the mixture, using two spoons, to the egg whites and top with a shrimp on each.
- Garnish with dill. You could also add capers for an additional bit of salty and sour goodness.

POACHED EGGS OVER ROASTED ASPARAGUS

Serves 2

Energy 167 kcal | Protein 16g | Fat 10g | Net Carbs 3.5g | P:E Ratio 1:1

Ingredients:

- 4 eggs
- 2 tbsp distilled white vinegar (optional)
- 1 bunch asparagus (about 16 spears)
- 2 tsp lemon juice
- 1/2 tsp ground black pepper
- 1/2 tsp garlic powder
- 2 tbsp fresh mixed herbs (parsley, mint, and thyme), chopped
- Pinch of sea salt

Instructions:

- Prepare the roasted asparagus. Preheat the oven to 450°F (230°C). Line the baking sheet with parchment paper. Trim off the hard end of each asparagus spear and arrange on the baking sheet. Drizzle lemon juice over asparagus. Season with salt, pepper, and garlic, and toss it to coat. Roast the asparagus for 8–10 minutes, shaking the sheet occasionally after 5 minutes to avoid overcooking. Move to the plate and top with herbs.

- Next, poach the eggs. Bring a large pot of water to boil. While waiting for the water to boil, crack an egg into a saucer and place a drop of vinegar in the water. Slide the egg into the water (the yolk should follow the white). Cook for 3–4 minutes. Remove the egg with a slotted spoon and dab it on a paper towel to remove any excess water.
- Place the eggs over asparagus. Season and serve immediately.

EGG SALAD LETTUCE WRAPS

Serves 2

Energy 163 kcal | Protein 18g | Fat 8g | Net Carbs 3.5g | P:E Ratio 1.5:1

Ingredients:

- 6 hard-boiled eggs (use only 3 yolks)
- 1/2 cup celery, chopped
- 1/4 cup red onion, finely diced
- 1/4 cup low-fat plain Greek yogurt (Two Good) (2.5 ounces)
- 1 tsp Dijon mustard
- 1/4 tsp smoked paprika
- 1/4 tsp ground black pepper
- 1 tbsp fresh dill, finely chopped
- 4 medium leaves of butter lettuce (or romaine lettuce)
- Pinch of sea salt

Instructions:

- Place the eggs in a pot and cover them with water. Place the pot over medium heat and bring to a light boil. Boil for 8–10 minutes to make sure the eggs are hardboiled. Remove the eggs from the pot and place in an ice bath or cold water for a few minutes before peeling.
- Chop eggs, celery, and red onion, and place everything in a bowl. Add in low-fat plain Greek yogurt, Dijon mustard, smoked paprika, ground black pepper, and fresh dill.
- Mix until well combined. Taste and season with salt. Serve in lettuce leaves.

FRIED EGGS WITH TURKEY AND SPINACH PLATE

Serves 2

Energy 271 kcal | Protein 55g | Fat 5g | Net Carbs 1g | P:E Ratio 9:1

Ingredients:

- 2 large eggs
- 12 oz turkey breast
- 2 cups fresh spinach
- 1/2 tsp dried mustard (optional)
- Pinch of sea salt and black pepper

Instructions:

- You can use one spray of nonstick olive oil or coconut oil cooking spray if you desire. Use a nontoxic, nonstick pan that will allow you to cook your eggs without sticking.
- Place the nonstick pan on a stove and let it heat perfectly over medium heat. Crack the egg into a small saucer and

pour into the pan. Sprinkle with salt and pepper. Cover the pan with the lid and cook for 2–3 minutes.
- When done, place the egg on a plate with turkey meat and spinach. Add dried mustard over spinach if desired.

CANADIAN BACON-WRAPPED EGG MUFFINS

Serves 2

Energy 230 kcal | Protein 24g | Fat 14g | Net Carbs 2g | P:E Ratio 1.5:1

Ingredients:

- 4 large eggs
- 4 oz Canadian bacon, thinly sliced
- Fresh basil for garnish (optional)
- Pinch of sea salt and black pepper

Instructions:

- Preheat the oven to 400°F (200°C). Use the standard-size muffin pan. Spray a piece of paper towel with nonstick olive oil or coconut oil cooking spray and wipe each well of the muffin pan.
- Line each well of the muffin pan (4) with a slice of Canadian bacon, making a bowl shape.
- Crack eggs into a bowl and whip. Pour egg into each cup (4) and season with salt and pepper.
- Bake for 12–14 minutes. Serve hot. Garnish with basil, if desired.

POULTRY-BASED RECIPES

SPICY CHICKEN CAKES

Serves 4

Energy 200 kcal | Protein 34.5g | Fat 5g | Net Carbs 1.5g | P:E Ratio 17:1

Ingredients:

- 3 cups shredded, cooked chicken meat
- 1 egg
- 1/4 red onion
- 1/2 red bell pepper
- 1 clove garlic, minced
- 1/4 jalapeño chili, seeds removed and finely chopped
- Pinch of sea salt and black pepper
- 2 tbsp chicken broth
- (2 tbsp ranchero sauce)

Instructions:

- Lightly sauté the onion, pepper, garlic, and jalapeño chili in a frying pan over medium heat until softened (approximately 5 minutes). Place the vegetables into a mixing bowl and let cool for a few minutes. Add the other ingredients to the bowl and mix everything together with your hands.
- Divide the mixture into 4 equal parts and mold it into balls. Press each ball between your hands to make 4 patties.
- Heat a large nonstick pan over medium-high heat and spray with olive oil or coconut oil cooking spray. Cook the chicken cakes for about 2–3 minutes on each side until golden brown.
- Serve hot or cold with a side of leafy greens or a salad.

CHICKEN SALAD-STUFFED ENDIVES

Serves 2

Energy 163 kcal | Protein 28g | Fat 3.5g | Net Carbs 2.5g | P:E Ratio 4.5:1

Ingredients:

- 2 chicken breasts, cooked
- 2 tbsp plain low-fat Greek yogurt (Two Good)
- 1 clove of garlic, minced
- 1/4 tsp chili paste
- 1/2 red bell pepper, finely diced
- 3 tbsp fresh cilantro, chopped
- 4 endive hearts
- Pinch of sea salt and black pepper

Instructions:

- Chop the cooked chicken breasts into small cubes and add them to a large mixing bowl. Add all other ingredients except the endive hearts. Mix together and season with salt and black pepper.
- Cut off the bases of the endives and discard a few of the large outside leaves. Wash the hearts well. Separate the leaves to use them. Using a spoon, fill each endive leaf with the chicken salad.
- Serve immediately on a plate.

LEMON PAN-COOKED CHICKEN BREASTS

Serves 2

Energy 198 kcal | Protein 26.5g | Fat 9g | Net Carbs 1.5g | P:E Ratio 2.5:1

Ingredients:

- 2 large chicken breasts
- 4 thin slices of lemon
- Zest of 1 lemon
- 4 cloves garlic, minced
- 1 tsp fresh thyme, chopped
- 1 tsp fresh oregano, chopped
- 1 tbsp olive oil
- Pinch of sea salt and black pepper

Instructions:

- Cut each chicken breast lengthwise into 2 pieces. Place the chicken breasts between 2 sheets of plastic wrap and use a rolling pin to pound the chicken breasts until they are 1/8 inch thick. Then use a fork to poke the chicken breasts to make the meat more tender.
- Sprinkle the meat with lemon zest, minced garlic, the freshly chopped herbs, and a small drizzle of olive oil. Rub the seasoning into chicken breasts with your hands.
- Add the remaining olive oil to a pan and heat. Once the oil is hot, add chicken breasts and cook for 5–7 minutes without moving them around. Flip the chicken breasts and cook for an additional 5–7 minutes or until fully cooked.
- Slice and serve with one slice of lemon and fresh herbs.

CHICKEN KABOBS AND VEGETABLES

Serves 2

Energy 115 kcal | Protein 15g | Fat 6g | Net Carbs 1g | P:E Ratio 2:1

Ingredients:

- 2 chicken thighs, skin removed, cut into chunks
- 2 cloves garlic, crushed
- 1 tbsp gluten-free tamari sauce

Instructions:

- Combine crushed garlic and tamari sauce in a bowl. Add chicken and toss until coated. Marinate for at least 2 hours or overnight.
- Preheat oven to 360°F (180°C). Thread chicken onto skewers and place in roasting tray. Bake for 30 minutes, turning after 15 minutes.
- Reserve any cooking juices at the end. Check to see if the chicken is cooked thoroughly.
- Serve on skewers and pour over the remaining marinade.

SPINACH-AND-MUSHROOM-STUFFED CHICKEN BREASTS

Serves 2

Energy 337 kcal | Protein 56g | Fat 9g | Net Carbs 5g | P:E Ratio 4:1

Ingredients:

- 4 boneless skinless chicken breasts
- 2 cups fresh spinach

- 2 garlic cloves, minced
- 1 cup mushrooms, finely chopped
- 1 tsp coconut oil
- 1/4 onion, diced
- 1/2 tsp red pepper flakes
- 1/4 cup white wine (optional)
- 1/2 cup chicken stock
- Pinch of sea salt and black pepper

Instructions:

- Cook the spinach in a large pan until wilted. Sprinkle with a pinch of salt. Squeeze out the water and move it to a bowl. Melt 1 tsp of coconut oil in a large skillet, and add the onion, garlic, and mushrooms. Cook for 3–5 minutes on medium heat. When it's done, add to the bowl with spinach and mix it all together.
- Make a horizontal cut through each of the chicken breasts to create a pocket. Stuff each breast with the spinach mixture and close the pockets with toothpicks.
- Sprinkle chicken breasts with salt, red pepper flakes, and black pepper evenly on both sides. Spray the skillet with olive oil or coconut oil cooking spray. Cook the chicken breasts over medium heat for about 4 minutes. Turn them over and add wine and stock to the pan. Cover the pan and cook for additional 5 minutes.
- Remove the lid and cook for another 2–4 minutes until the chicken is done.

ROASTED CHICKEN AND VEGGIES BOWL

Serves 2

Energy 215 kcal | Protein 30g | Fat 6g | Net Carbs 8g | P:E Ratio 2:1

Ingredients:

- 2 chicken breasts, chopped
- 1 cup bell pepper, chopped
- 1/2 white onion, chopped
- 1 zucchini, chopped
- 1 cup broccoli florets
- 1 tsp olive oil
- 1 tsp Italian seasoning
- 1/4 tsp paprika (optional)
- Pinch of sea salt and black pepper

Instructions:

- Preheat oven to 400°F (200°C). Chop the vegetables into big chunks. Chop the chicken breasts into cubes. Mix the vegetables and the chicken together in a medium roasting dish or sheet pan. Add the olive oil, salt, pepper, Italian seasoning, and paprika. Toss to combine.
- Bake in the oven for about 25 minutes until the chicken is cooked. Serve hot.

CHINESE DRUMSTICKS WITH FRESH CUCUMBER SALAD

Serves 4

Energy 193 kcal | Protein 21g | Fat 9.5g | Net Carbs 6.5g | P:E Ratio 1.5:1

Ingredients:

- 8 chicken drumsticks
- 2 garlic cloves, peeled and crushed
- 1 tsp sesame oil
- 4 tbsp gluten-free tamari
- 2 tsp five-spice powder*
- 2 medium cucumbers
- 1/8 cup fresh dill
- 1/2 red onion
- 1/8 cup white wine vinegar
- 1/8 cup water
- Pinch of sea salt and black pepper
- 1 tsp sesame seeds

Instructions:

- In a large bowl, mix together the five-spice powder, tamari, sesame oil, and garlic. Slice each drumstick through the thickest part 2–3 times and put in the marinade. Mix well, cover, and leave in the refrigerator for at least 30 minutes.
- Preheat the oven to 400°F (200°C). Cover a large baking tray with foil. Place the drumsticks on the tray and bake for 15–20 minutes. Remove from the oven. Brush the chicken with the remaining marinade and return to the oven for another 10–15 minutes or until chicken is cooked.
- Slice the cucumbers in thin rounds. Slice the onion in thin strips. In a medium bowl, mix the cucumbers, onion, and

fresh dill. Season with salt and pepper. Mix together white wine vinegar and water. Pour it over the cucumber mix and stir well. Add salt and pepper to taste.

- Serve the chicken with cucumber salad and garnish with sesame seeds.

*For five-spice powder, I recommend Simply Organic, which contains organic cinnamon, organic fennel seed, organic cloves, organic star anise, and organic white pepper.

CUCUMBER CHICKEN MEATWICH

Serves 2

Energy 154 kcal | Protein 27g | Fat 3g | Net Carbs 3g | P:E Ratio 4.5:1

Ingredients:

- 2 chicken breasts as "bread"
- 2 tbsp apple cider vinegar
- 4 cups cucumber, sliced
- 1 tbsp dill
- 1 tbsp fresh parsley, chopped
- 1 tbsp green onion, chopped
- 2 tsp lemon juice
- 1 tsp garlic powder
- 1 tsp tarragon
- Pinch of sea salt and black pepper

Instructions:

- Put the apple cider vinegar, cucumbers, dill, parsley, green onion, lemon juice, salt, pepper, garlic powder, and tarragon into a bowl and toss together. Set aside to marinate.

- Pound the chicken breasts to be as thin as possible (about 1/4 inch). Slice into "bread" sizes (if you had two whole chicken breasts, pound and then slice each in half, giving you 4 pieces).
- Season chicken with salt and pepper and grill for about three minutes. Flip and grill for two more minutes. Assemble the chicken sandwiches with grilled chicken as bread and marinated cucumber slices inside. Drizzle any extra cucumber marinade over the top of the sandwich.
- Serve with additional cucumber salad on the side. Enjoy while the chicken is hot or chilled.

TURKEY LETTUCE FAJITAS

Serves 4

Energy 152 kcal | Protein 20g | Fat 3.5g | Net Carbs 8.5g | P:E Ratio 1.5:1

Ingredients:

- 12–14 oz turkey breast steaks, cut into thin strips
- 3.5 oz low-fat plain Greek yogurt (Two Good)
- 8 iceberg lettuce leaves, washed and dried
- 1 tsp olive oil
- 1 medium red onion
- 2 bell peppers (1 red and 1 yellow)
- 1 tsp smoked paprika
- 1 tsp ground cumin
- 1 tsp ground coriander
- Pinch of sea salt and black pepper
- 8 lime wedges

Instructions:

- Cut off the stalk end of the lettuce and separate the leaves. Peel away at least eight leaves. Wash and dry them well. Place the leaves on a serving plate.
- Heat the olive oil in a large pan over medium heat. Cook together the turkey, onion, and peppers for 5–6 minutes or until the turkey is cooked and the vegetables are softened. Add the spices and cook for another 1–2 minutes, stirring.
- Season with salt and freshly ground pepper. Fill the lettuce leaves with the hot turkey mixture. Top with Greek yogurt, and serve with lime wedges.

TURKEY MEATBALLS

Serves 4

Energy 283 kcal | Protein 32.5g | Fat 16g | Net Carbs 0.5g | P:E Ratio 2:1

Ingredients:

- 1 pound ground turkey
- 1 egg, large
- 1/2 cup shredded zucchini, liquid squeezed out (measured before squeezing)
- 2 large garlic cloves, grated
- 1 tbsp onion flakes or powder
- 1/2 tsp dried oregano
- 1/2 tsp salt
- Ground black pepper, to taste

Instructions:

- Preheat the oven to 375°F (190°C). Line a large baking sheet with parchment paper and spray with olive oil or coconut oil cooking spray.
- In a large bowl, add all the ingredients together and mix well with your hands.
- Using a small scoop, form the meatballs and lay them on the baking sheet. Bake the meatballs for fifteen minutes. Then turn and toss with a spatula and bake for five more minutes. Serve hot.

TURKEY LETTUCE WRAPS

Serves 4

Energy 278 kcal | Protein 31.5g | Fat 15g | Net Carbs 1.5g | P:E Ratio 2:1

Ingredients:

- 1 lb ground turkey
- 1 medium zucchini
- 2 cloves garlic, minced
- 2 tbsp curry powder
- 1/4 tsp chili paste
- 1/2 cup water
- 1 chicken stock cube or 1 tsp chicken bouillon paste
- 8 large romaine lettuce leaves, washed and dried
- Pinch of sea salt and black pepper

Instructions:

- Slice the zucchini into thin half-rounds and cook over medium heat for about 5 minutes. Add the garlic and cook for another minute. Remove from the pan and set aside.

- Place the turkey in the same pan over medium-high heat. When the turkey starts to brown, after about 5 minutes, add the curry powder and the chili paste.
- Cook for another 3–5 minutes, until the meat is fully cooked. Add zucchini, water, and chicken bullion, and bring to a boil.
- When it starts to boil, reduce the heat and continue to cook for another 10 minutes until the water has evaporated. Remove from the heat.
- Fill the lettuce leaves with the turkey mixture and serve immediately.

BEEF-BASED RECIPES
BASIL BURGER ON LEAFY GREENS

Serves 2

Energy 250 kcal | Protein 30g | Fat 12g | Net Carbs 2.5g | P:E Ratio 2:1

Ingredients:

- 8 oz lean ground beef (90 percent lean)
- 4 tsp coconut aminos
- 1 tsp dried basil or 2 fresh basil leaves, finely chopped
- 1/4 tsp garlic salt
- 1/8 tsp ground black pepper
- 1 cup mixed leafy greens

Instructions:

- In a medium bowl, combine all ingredients and mix well with your hands. Form 4 small burger patties.
- Grill for about 3 minutes on each side or until fully cooked.
- Serve with mixed leafy greens.

SPINACH AND MUSHROOM MEATBALLS

Serves 8

Energy 272 kcal | Protein 32g | Fat 14g | Net Carbs 1g | P:E Ratio 2:1

Ingredients:

- 2 lbs high-quality ground beef
- 1 egg
- 1/2 small onion, finely chopped
- 3 cloves garlic
- 1 tbsp olive oil
- 1 large portobello mushroom, finely diced
- 8 oz fresh spinach
- 1/4 tsp smoked paprika
- 1 tbsp fresh oregano, chopped
- 1 tbsp fresh thyme, chopped
- 1 tbsp fresh parsley, chopped
- 1 tbsp fresh sage, chopped
- Pinch of sea salt and black pepper

Instructions:

- Preheat the oven to 400°F. Line a deep baking sheet with parchment paper.
- Sauté onion and garlic in a pan with a little olive oil until soft. Add the mushroom and chopped fresh spinach. Season with salt and pepper and cook over medium heat for 5–8 minutes.
- Place the cooked veggies into a strainer over an empty bowl and let sit for 5 minutes to get rid of any excess juices. Press the veggies to remove any remaining moisture before placing into a large mixing bowl.
- Add the ground beef, seasoning, chopped herbs, and egg to

the mixing bowl with veggies. Use your hands to mix the ingredients together. Once mixed well, make 16 meatballs. Use 3–4 tablespoons of the mixture and roll into balls.

- Place the meatballs onto the baking sheet and drizzle with a little olive oil. Place in the oven and bake for 35 minutes, turning halfway through.

HOMEMADE JERKY

Serves 4

Energy 234 kcal | Protein 42g | Fat 6g | Net Carbs 1g | P:E Ratio 6:1

Ingredients:

- 1 lb grass-fed beef top round, fat removed
- 1/4 cup gluten-free tamari
- 1 tsp onion powder
- 1 tsp smoked paprika
- 3/4 tsp chili powder
- 1/2 tsp garlic powder
- 1/2 tsp sea salt

Instructions:

- Place the meat in the freezer for 2 hours to make slicing easier. Slice the beef as thin as possible, into about 1/8-inch-thick pieces.
- In a medium bowl, combine all the remaining ingredients. Add the meat and toss until well combined. Cover and refrigerate for 12–24 hours. Make sure you flip the meat at least once while marinating to evenly cover the pieces.
- Preheat the oven to 150F. Line two baking sheets with parch-

ment paper. Remove the meat from marinade. Drain well and pat dry with a paper towel. Place the meat slices on the baking sheets. Make sure the pieces don't touch.

- Place in the oven and cook until dry to the touch (up to 8 hours depending on the thickness). Remember to flip the slices every hour or so to make sure they dry evenly.
- Once fully dry, remove from the oven and allow to cool completely. Store in an airtight container at room temperature for up to 2 months.

BEEF-STUFFED CELERY STICKS

Serves 2

Energy 287 kcal | Protein 33g | Fat 12g | Net Carbs 6.5g | P:E Ratio 2:1

Ingredients:

- 8 oz grass-fed ground beef (90 percent lean)
- 2 tsp minced garlic
- 2 tbsp minced ginger
- 1 tsp five-spice blend
- 1 tbsp coconut aminos
- 1 tbsp rice vinegar
- 4–8 long celery stalks
- 1/4 cup green onions, thinly sliced
- Pinch of sea salt and black pepper

Instructions:

- Sauté the beef, garlic, and ginger over medium-high heat for 2–3 minutes, until ginger and garlic are softened. Reduce heat to low. Season with salt, pepper, and five-spice blend.

- Stir in coconut aminos and rice vinegar and continue cooking for about 5 minutes.
- Stuff the celery stalks with the beef mixture and garnish with sliced green onions.

TACO SALAD

Serves 2

Energy 289 kcal | Protein 33g | Fat 12g | Net Carbs 6g | P:E Ratio 2:1

Ingredients:

- 8 oz grass-fed ground beef (90 percent lean)
- 1.5 tsp chili powder
- 1/8 tsp garlic powder
- 1/8 tsp onion powder
- 1/8 tsp dried oregano
- 1/4 tsp paprika
- 1/2 tsp ground cumin
- 1/2 cup tomato, chopped
- 1/2 cup green onions, chopped
- 4 cups iceberg lettuce, chopped
- Pinch of sea salt and black pepper

Dressing

- 1/4 cup apple cider vinegar
- 1 tbsp lime juice
- 6 tablespoons sugar-free salsa
- Pinch of sea salt and black pepper

Instructions:

- In a small bowl, combine all the dry seasoning for the ground beef.
- Place ground beef in a large skillet and place over medium heat. Break the beef apart into small crumbles while cooking. Add seasoning mix to the skillet and stir to combine. Cook ground beef for about 8 minutes or until all the juice has evaporated and beef is browned nicely. Stir occasionally and set aside once it's cooked.
- In a small bowl, combine all the ingredients for the dressing and whisk together.
- Place chopped lettuce, tomato, and green onion in a large bowl. Pour the dressing over the salad mix and toss. Divide the salad between two bowls and top each with half of the cooked ground beef.

ZUCCHINI LASAGNA

Serves 2

Energy 279 kcal | Protein 31.5g | Fat 12g | Net Carbs 3.5g | P:E Ratio 2:1

Ingredients:

- 8 oz grass-fed ground beef (90 percent lean)
- 2 medium zucchinis
- 1/2 cup canned tomatoes
- 1 tsp dried basil
- 1 tsp minced garlic
- 1 tbsp onion, finely chopped
- 1.5 tsp nutritional yeast
- 2 tbsp fat-free beef broth
- Pinch of sea salt and black pepper

Instructions:

- Slice zucchini horizontally using a mandolin slicer to create very thin, long "lasagna" noodles. Set the noodles aside.
- Sauté ground beef in 1 tbsp beef broth, sea salt, and black pepper in a pan. Cook over medium heat and break up the ground beef while stirring so there are no large clumps. Set aside.
- Add 1 tbsp beef broth, garlic, and onions to a small pan and sauté until garlic begins to brown. Add canned tomatoes, basil, 1/4 tsp black pepper, and 1/2 tsp salt to the pan. Bring to a boil. Boil for 3–5 minutes or until slightly thick. Remove from heat and puree.
- Add cooked ground beef to sauce and spread a thin layer in the bottom of a small casserole dish (8-inch square pan is ideal). Place a layer of zucchini slices in the bottom of the pan on top of the sauce, covering the whole bottom. Scoop about 1/3 of the sauce on top of the zucchini and spread evenly. Add another layer of zucchini slices on top of the sauce. Repeat until you have used all the sauce and zucchini.
- Bake at 350°F (180°C) for 20 minutes or until sauce is bubbling around the sides of the pan. Sprinkle lasagna with nutritional yeast and serve.

MEATZA

Serves 2

Energy 316 kcal | Protein 34g | Fat 12g | Net Carbs 11g | P:E Ratio 1.5:1

Ingredients:

- 8 oz grass-fed lean ground beef (90 percent lean)

- 3/4 cup red bell pepper, sliced
- 3/4 cup green bell pepper, sliced
- 1/2 cup red onion, sliced
- 4 oz button mushrooms, sliced
- 1 tsp garlic, minced
- 1 tsp fresh parsley, chopped
- 1 tsp fresh basil, chopped
- 1 tsp fresh oregano, chopped
- 2 tbsp tomato paste
- 1 tbsp water
- Pinch of sea salt

Instructions:

- Preheat the oven to 450°F. Line a rimmed baking sheet with parchment paper.
- In a medium bowl, combine ground beef, garlic, and half the fresh spices/herbs and salt. Using your hands, mix until well combined.
- Add the beef mixture to the baking sheet and flatten into a round, thin circle. Wrap a wooden rolling pin with parchment paper and gently roll out the meat. Try not to tear the meat. Bake the "crust" for 10 minutes. Remove the baking sheet from the oven. Use a paper towel to soak up the juices before flipping the crust. Reduce temperature to 350°F. Bake an additional 10 minutes.
- While the pizza crust is baking, stir together tomato paste and water. Remove the pizza crust from the oven. Top the pizza with tomato paste mixture. Sprinkle over bell peppers, red onion, and mushrooms. Return to the oven for approximately 5–8 minutes, until the vegetables are crisp and tender.
- Sprinkle with remaining fresh herbs. Serve immediately.

SLOPPY JOE LETTUCE WRAPS

Serves 2

Energy 293 kcal | Protein 34g | Fat 12g | Net Carbs 7.5g | P:E Ratio 2:1

Ingredients:

- 8 oz grass-fed ground beef (90 percent lean)
- 1/2 cup white onion, minced
- 2 tbsp green onion, minced
- 2/3 cup celery, minced
- 2 tsp garlic, minced
- 1/2 tsp cayenne pepper
- 1/2 tbsp white vinegar
- 2 tbsp tomato paste
- 4 oz button mushrooms, minced
- 1/4 cup red bell pepper, minced
- 2 cups butter lettuce leaves
- Pinch of sea salt

Instructions:

- Be sure to chop all the vegetables finely, using a chopper or a food processor.
- Heat a large skillet over medium-high heat. Add meat to the skillet, breaking it up as it cooks. Season with cayenne pepper. Cook until meat browns. Add onion, green onion, celery, garlic, mushrooms, and red bell pepper. Reduce heat to medium. Add white vinegar and cook for 5 minutes.
- Add tomato paste, stirring to combine well. Cover and reduce to a simmer. Cook for an additional 5 minutes.
- Serve approximately 1/3 cup of the sloppy joe mixture on each leaf of butter lettuce.

MEATBALLS WITH GARLIC SPINACH

Serves 2

Energy 276 kcal | Protein 34.5g | Fat 12g | Net Carbs 3g | P:E Ratio 2:1

Ingredients:

- 8 oz grass-fed ground beef (90 percent lean)
- 1 egg white
- 1/4 cup fat-free beef broth (or water)
- 1/2 cup tomato sauce
- 1/2 cup water
- 2 tbsp onion
- 1/4 tsp dried parsley
- 1/2 tsp garlic powder
- 1/8 tsp dried mustard powder
- 4 cups baby spinach
- 1/2 tsp minced garlic
- Pinch of sea salt

Instructions:

- In a large bowl, combine ground beef, egg white, onion, parsley, garlic powder, mustard powder, and salt. Knead together with your hands and divide into meatballs (10–12 meatballs).
- In a large skillet, heat beef broth and add meatballs to the hot pan. Sear over medium-high heat and rotate meatballs several times to brown them on each side. Once cooked, transfer meatballs and remaining broth into a slow cooker.
- Pour the sauce and water into a slow cooker. Set on low and cook for 4 hours. Place baby spinach in a large skillet with 1/4 cup water and garlic. Cover and steam for 4 minutes or until wilted. Serve alongside the meatballs.

PORTOBELLO BEEF BURGER

Serves 2

Energy 283 kcal | Protein 34.5g | Fat 12.5g | Net Carbs 5g | P:E Ratio 2:1

Ingredients:

- 8 oz grass-fed ground beef (90 percent lean)
- 2 medium portobello mushroom caps
- 1/4 cup white onion, thinly sliced
- 1/4 tsp garlic powder
- 1 tsp balsamic vinegar
- 2 tsp Dijon mustard
- 2 large lettuce leaves
- Pinch of sea salt and black pepper

Instructions:

- Heat a small pan over medium-high heat. Spray with olive oil or coconut oil cooking spray and sauté the sliced onions until golden brown. Remove from heat and set aside.
- Combine the ground beef, salt, pepper, garlic powder, and balsamic vinegar in a bowl and mix until well combined. Divide into two equal portions and shape into patties. Remove the gills from the portobello mushroom caps.
- Preheat grill or grill pan to medium-high heat. Spray grates with nonstick cooking spray. Cook the burgers for about 5 minutes on each side (for medium-well) and the portobello mushroom caps for about 4 minutes on each side, until slightly softened. Top each burger with the sautéed onions, a lettuce leaf, and 1 tsp Dijon mustard.
- Serve on a mushroom cap.

PORK-BASED RECIPES

BACON AND VEGGIES FRY-UP

Serves 2

Energy 176 kcal | Protein 9g | Fat 6g | Net Carbs 5.5g | P:E Ratio 1:1.25

Ingredients:

- 4 strips of bacon
- 1 cup raw broccoli, cut into small florets
- 1 cup chestnut mushrooms, sliced
- 10 cherry tomatoes, halved
- 1 tbsp olive oil
- Pinch of black pepper

Instructions:

- Fill a saucepan with the water to 1/3 and bring to a boil. Add the broccoli. Cook for three minutes and then drain.
- Heat the oil in a large nonstick pan. Cook the bacon, mushrooms, and tomatoes for 2 minutes, or until the mushrooms are lightly browned. Add the broccoli and cook for one more minute.
- Season with black pepper. Divide between two plates and serve immediately.

PERFECT PULLED PORK

Serves 4

Energy 328 kcal | Protein 34.5g | Fat 18g | Net Carbs 5g | P:E Ratio 1.5:1

Ingredients:

- 2 pounds pork shoulder joint with fat removed
- 3 tbsp tomato puree
- 2 tbsp chipotle paste
- Juice of one orange
- Juice of 2 limes
- 1 tsp ground cumin
- 1 tsp ground allspice
- Pinch of sea salt and black pepper

Instructions:

- Prepare the marinade. Whisk together in a large bowl the tomato puree, chipotle paste, orange and lime juice, salt, and spices.
- Remove any string from the pork and add the meat to the marinade. Turn the pork several times until well coated. Cover and put in the refrigerator to marinate for at least 8 hours.
- Preheat the oven to 340F. Place the pork and the marinade in a medium casserole. Cover, and bake for about 3 hours, or until the pork falls apart when prodded with a fork. Check after 1.5 hours and add a little extra water if needed.
- Transfer the pork to a warmed large platter and shred with two forks, discarding the rind and fat. Can be served in lettuce wraps or with a side of homemade coleslaw.

GREEN BEAN HAM SALAD

Serves 2

Energy 230 kcal | Protein 28g | Fat 3g | Net Carbs 17g | P:E Ratio 1.5:1

Ingredients:

- 8 oz extra lean ham, cooked, cubed
- 4 cups green beans, trimmed into 2–3-inch pieces
- 1 cup white onion, sliced
- 1/2 tsp dried oregano
- 2 tbsp roasted garlic, smashed
- 2 tbsp balsamic vinegar
- Pinch of sea salt and black pepper

Instructions:

- Add 4 tbsp water to a large skillet along with the onion slices. Cook over medium heat, stirring occasionally until the water has evaporated and the onions are beginning to brown on the bottom of the pan (about 8 minutes).
- Add another 4 tbsp of water to the pan along with oregano and let the water cook off again, stirring occasionally. The onions should be nicely browned and caramelized. Blend the roasted garlic, vinegar, salt, and pepper in a small bowl to make the dressing.
- Bring a small saucepan of water (about 6 quarts) to a boil. Add green beans and boil for 2 minutes. Strain and place in a bowl of ice water to stop the cooking process.
- Toss green beans together with the onion mix and the garlic dressing. Serve and enjoy!

PORK STIR-FRY

Serves 2

Energy 264 kcal | Protein 31.5g | Fat 10g | Net Carbs 6.5g | P:E Ratio 2:1

Ingredients:

- 8 oz pork tenderloin (fillet), trimmed, cut into slices
- 1 pack (16 oz) stir-fry vegetables
- 1 tbsp olive oil
- 2–3 tbsp fresh root ginger, pilled and finely grated
- 1 tsp almond flour
- 1 tbsp gluten-free tamari
- 1/4 tsp crushed dried chili flakes
- Pinch of sea salt and black pepper

Instructions:

- Season the pork loin with sea salt and black pepper.
- Heat the oil in a large nonstick pan or wok over medium-high heat. Add the pork and stir-fry, tossing frequently, for 3–4 minutes. Add the vegetables and stir-fry with the pork for another 2–3 minutes. Add the ginger and toss.
- Mix together in a small bowl the almond flour, tamari, and chili flakes. Stir into the pan and toss everything together for 1–2 minutes.
- Serve immediately with a little extra tamari if desired.

FISH- AND SEAFOOD-BASED RECIPES
COD STEAKS WITH BROCCOLI

Serves 2

Energy 207 kcal | Protein 30.5g | Fat 2g | Net Carbs 12.5g | P:E Ratio 2:1

Ingredients:

- 8 ounces thick skinless cod fillets
- 1 bunch broccoli
- 1/2 tsp crushed dried chili flakes
- 1 tbsp nutritional yeast
- Olive oil or coconut oil cooking spray
- Pinch of sea salt and black pepper

Instructions:

- Cut the broccoli crowns off the stems and break the crowns up into smaller florets.
- Bring about 1 inch of water to boil in a saucepan with a steamer. Add the broccoli to the steamer and cover. Reduce the heat and steam for 5–6 minutes. As soon as the broccoli softens, remove from heat and place on a serving plate. Sprinkle with a pinch of sea salt and a tablespoon of nutritional yeast.
- Season the cod fillets with salt and pepper on both sides. Spray the preheated nonstick pan with the cooking spray. Add the cod fillets and cook for about 4 minutes. Flip the fish and sprinkle with some chili flakes. Cook on the other side for another 3–5 minutes. The cod is ready when it is just beginning to flake into large chunks.
- Serve hot with a side of steamed broccoli.

SEARED SCALLOPS WITH CAULIFLOWER RICE

Serves 2

Energy 218 kcal | Protein 21g | Fat 6.5g | Net Carbs 13g | P:E Ratio 1:1

Ingredients:

- 12 large sea scallops
- 1 head cauliflower (or 1 pound riced cauliflower)
- 2 tbsp fresh parsley leaves
- 1 tbsp olive or avocado oil
- Juice of 1/2 lemon
- 1/2 medium onion
- Pinch of sea salt and black pepper

Instructions:

- Cut off the stems of cauliflower as much as possible. Break up the florets into a food processor and pulse until the mixture looks like rice. You can chop the cauliflower with a knife as well or simply use riced cauliflower from the store.
- Chop the onion into small pieces. Heat the oil in a large nonstick pan over medium-high heat. Add the onions and cook, stirring frequently, until the onions are golden brown and have softened (approximately 8 minutes). Add the cauliflower and stir well to combine. Add the salt and continue to cook, stirring frequently, for about 3–5 minutes.
- Remove from heat and put in a large serving bowl. Garnish with parsley, sprinkle with lemon juice, and season to taste with salt. Serve warm.
- Pat the scallops dry and sprinkle with the sea salt and black pepper. Heat olive or avocado oil in a large sauté pan over high heat. Once hot, add scallops and cook for 2 minutes.

Then flip to the other side and cook for another 2–3 minutes, until golden brown.

- Remove to a paper towel and serve on the cauliflower rice.

SALMON BURGERS WITH GREEN MASH

Serves 4

Energy 447 kcal | Protein 43g | Fat 25g | Net Carbs 7.5g | P:E Ratio 1.5:1

Ingredients:

- 24 oz salmon
- 1 egg
- 1 head broccoli
- 1/2 yellow onion
- 1 tbsp olive or avocado oil
- Pinch of sea salt and black pepper

Instructions:

- Cut the salmon into small pieces and place in a food processor together with the ingredients for the burgers. Pulse for 30–45 seconds until you have a smooth mixture. Shape 6–8 burgers.
- Preheat the olive or avocado oil on medium heat and cook the burgers for 4–5 minutes per side.
- Trim the broccoli and cut into small florets. You can use the stem as well; peel it and chop into small pieces. Bring a pot of lightly salted water to a boil and add the broccoli. Cook for a few minutes to soften.
- Use a blender or a food processor to turn the broccoli into a green mash. Season with salt and pepper. Serve with warm salmon burgers.

GINGER BAKED FISH OVER FRESH GREENS

Serves 2

Energy 211 kcal | Protein 23g | Fat 7g | Net Carbs 10g | P:E Ratio 1.5:1

Ingredients:

- 8 oz thick white fish fillet, such as cod
- 4 cups mixed fresh greens, such as spinach, kale, and arugula
- 1 onion, sliced
- 1 tbsp olive oil
- 1 garlic clove, peeled and thinly sliced
- 2–3 tbsp fresh root ginger, pilled and finely grated
- 1/4 tsp crushed dried chili flakes
- Juice of 1/2 lime
- Pinch of sea salt and black pepper

Instructions:

- Preheat the oven to 400°F. Cover a baking tray with foil and drizzle with olive oil. Place the fish on one half of the foil, leaving enough to cover.
- Sprinkle the fish with garlic, ginger, onion, and chili flakes, and squeeze the lime juice over the fish. Season with sea salt and black pepper. Then fold the foil over the fish to cover. Bake the fish for 12–15 minutes.
- Cover the serving plate with the greens and place the fish on top. Spoon the cooking juices from the foil over the fish and greens and serve.

TUNA LETTUCE CUPS

Serves 2

Energy 221 kcal | Protein 39g | Fat 2g | Net Carbs 6g | P:E Ratio 5:1

Ingredients:

- 10 oz no-drain canned tuna
- 1/2 small red onion, very thinly sliced
- 5 cherry tomatoes
- 1 romaine lettuce heart
- Pinch of sea salt and black pepper

Instructions:

- Set aside 6 romaine leaves for cups.
- Chop the smaller leaves and put in a bowl. Add the tuna, onion, and tomatoes. Season with salt and pepper, and mix well.
- Fill up the lettuce cups with the tuna mixture and serve.

EDAMAME TUNA SALAD

Serves 2

Energy 340 kcal | Protein 49g | Fat 7g | Net Carbs 12.5g | P:E Ratio 2.5:1

Ingredients:

- 10 oz no-drain, canned tuna
- 8 oz frozen edamame beans
- 1 spring onion, trimmed and thinly sliced
- Fresh parsley leaves, chopped

- 1.5 tbsp apple cider vinegar
- 2 cups mixed greens, chopped
- Pinch of sea salt and pepper

Instructions:

- Thaw the frozen beans by covering them with just-boiled water for 1 minute. Drain and rinse with cold water.
- Place the tuna in a bowl and break into small flakes with the fork. Add the beans, spring onions, and parsley leaves and drizzle with vinegar. Sprinkle with salt and pepper and mix together well.
- Add the chopped, mixed greens right before serving.

GRILLED SHRIMP AND ZUCCHINI

Serves 2

Energy 291 kcal | Protein 48g | Fat 8.5g | Net Carbs 2g | P:E Ratio 4.5:1

Ingredients:

- 1 lb peeled jumbo shrimp
- 1 medium zucchini
- 1 tbsp olive oil
- 2 tbsp lemon juice
- 1 tbsp smoked paprika
- 1 tsp garlic powder
- 1 tsp onion powder
- 1 tsp dried oregano
- 1 tsp dried basil
- 1/4 tsp cayenne pepper
- Pinch of sea salt and black pepper

Instructions:

- Place the shrimp into a large mixing bowl. Drizzle with olive oil and lemon juice.
- Sprinkle paprika, garlic powder, onion powder, oregano, basil, salt, pepper, and cayenne pepper over shrimp. Toss to coat. Cover and refrigerate while preparing the zucchini.
- Slice the zucchini into thin circles. Sprinkle with sea salt and pepper.
- Preheat grill to high heat, about 400°F. Soak wooden skewers in water for 10 minutes.
- Thread shrimp and zucchini onto skewers to cook, or place directly on the grill individually. Cook for 2–3 minutes per side. Serve hot.

SALMON WITH PESTO AND SPINACH

Serves 4

Energy 384 kcal | Protein 42g | Fat 22g | 2.5g Net Carbs | P:E Ratio 2:1

Ingredients:

- 24 oz salmon
- 1 cup plain low-fat Greek yogurt (Two Good)
- 1 lb fresh spinach
- 1 tbsp green or red pesto
- 1 tsp olive oil
- Pinch of sea salt and black pepper

Instructions:

- Preheat the oven to 400°F (200°C). Spray the baking dish

with olive oil or coconut oil cooking spray. Season the salmon fillets with salt and pepper and place them in the prepared baking dish.

- Mix Greek yogurt and pesto and spread over the salmon. Bake for 15–20 minutes, or until the salmon is cooked through and flakes easily with a fork.
- Sauté the spinach in olive oil until it's wilted, about 2 minutes. Season with salt and pepper. Serve immediately with the oven-baked salmon.

BROILED SALMON WITH MUSTARD GLAZE

Serves 4

Energy 350 kcal | Protein 17g | Fat 22g | Net Carbs 1g | P:E Ratio 1.5:1

Ingredients:

- 4 six-ounce salmon fillets
- 4 lemon wedges
- 2 garlic cloves
- 3/4 tsp fresh rosemary leaves, finely chopped
- 3/4 tsp fresh thyme leaves, finely chopped
- 1 tbsp dry white wine
- 1 tsp extra-virgin olive oil
- 2 tbsp Dijon mustard
- 2 tbsp whole-grain mustard
- Pinch of sea salt and black pepper

Instructions:

- In a food processor, combine garlic, rosemary, thyme, wine, oil, Dijon mustard, and 1 tbsp of whole-grain mustard. Blend the sauce until combined, about 30 seconds. Transfer to a small bowl. Add the remaining 1 tbsp of whole-grain mustard to the sauce and stir to combine. Set aside.

- Preheat the broiler. Line a baking sheet with foil. Spray the foil with olive oil or coconut oil cooking spray. Arrange the salmon fillets on the baking sheet and sprinkle with salt and pepper. Broil for 2 minutes.
- Spoon the mustard sauce over the fillets. Continue broiling until the fillets are cooked through and golden brown, about 5 minutes longer.
- Transfer the fillets to plates and serve with lemon wedges.

BACON-WRAPPED SHRIMP

Serves 4

Energy 208 kcal | Protein 31g | Fat 7g | Net Carbs 1g | P:E Ratio 4:1

Ingredients:

- 1 lb (30–35 count) raw peeled shrimp
- 12–15 strips hickory-smoked bacon, cut in half
- 1 tsp olive oil
- Zest from 1 lime
- 2 tbsp lime juice
- 1 tsp chili powder (more or less to taste)

Instructions:

- Prepare grill on high, direct heat (if grilling) or preheat oven to 400°F (200°C). If grilling and using thin bamboo or wood skewers, soak them in water first for 30 minutes.
- Mix together in a small bowl the lime zest, lime juice, olive

oil, and chili powder. Stir the shrimp into the lime-chili mixture. Make sure each piece is well coated.

- Spread the bacon pieces out over several layers of paper towels on a microwave-safe plate. Cover with another layer of paper towel. Microwave on high until the bacon fat begins to melt but the bacon is still somewhat pliable, about 1–2 minutes.
- Wrap a half piece of partially cooked bacon around each piece of shrimp. If you are grilling, thread the shrimp onto skewers. If you are using the oven, secure each bacon strip onto the shrimp with toothpicks.
- Place the bacon-wrapped shrimp on a foil-lined baking pan. Brush the remaining lime-chili mixture on the outside of the bacon-wrapped shrimp. Grill uncovered for 3 minutes on each side (less or more time depending on the heat of your grill) or bake in the 400°F (200°C) oven for 8–10 minutes, or until the bacon is lightly browned and the shrimp is cooked through.

GINGER SCALLOPS

Serves 2

Energy 246 kcal | Protein 22g | Fat 13g | Net Carbs 10g | P:E Ratio 1:1

Ingredients:

- 8 oz scallops (10–12 large scallops)
- 8 cups baby spinach
- 2 cups shiitake mushrooms, sliced
- 1/2 cup carrot ginger miso dressing (Trader Joe's)
- 2 tbsp fresh cilantro, chopped
- 1/4 cup green onions, chopped

- 6 oz Miracle Noodles
- Pinch of sea salt and black pepper

Instructions:

- Heat a large skillet over medium heat and add dressing and green onions. Sprinkle scallops with the salt and then cook scallops for 1–2 minutes on each side. Remove from pan and set aside.
- Add the spinach and mushrooms to the skillet and cover, allowing vegetables to cook for about 3–4 minutes, stirring occasionally. Toss spinach and mushrooms with Miracle Noodles and place scallops on top. Garnish with fresh cilantro and serve.

PLANT-BASED RECIPES
TOFU STIR FRY

Serves 2

Energy 275 kcal | Protein 26.5g | Fat 15.5g | Net Carbs 7.5g | P:E Ratio 1:1

Ingredients:

- 16 oz firm tofu
- 16 oz asparagus
- 1 tbsp gluten-free tamari
- 1 tbsp green onions, finely chopped
- 2 tsp red chili sauce
- 2 tsp olive or avocado oil

Sauce

- 3 tbsp gluten-free tamari
- 1 tbsp sesame oil
- 1.5 tbsp rice vinegar
- 5 cloves garlic, minced
- 1/2 tbsp ginger, freshly grated
- 1/2 cup water

Instructions:

- Cut the block of tofu in half. Place each half in 2 clean paper towels, one at a time, and gently press/squeeze to remove excess stored liquid (without breaking up the tofu). Cut the tofu into 1/2-inch cubes and pan-cook on medium-high heat in a nonstick pan with 1 tsp of olive or avocado oil. Mix and turn frequently until all the water is burned off and the tofu is lightly golden brown all around (be careful not to burn the tofu).
- Once the tofu is cooked, add 1 tbsp tamari and toss once more. Set the tofu aside.
- Whisk all the sauce ingredients in a small bowl and set aside.
- Trim the bottom of the asparagus spears and cut them into 2-inch-long pieces. For other vegetables, dice them to the preferred size.
- Heat 1 tsp of olive or avocado oil on medium-high heat. Add in the diced veggies and sauté until cooked through but still slightly crispy. Add in the cooked tofu and sauce. Turn the heat down to medium and let it simmer.
- Taste and adjust flavor if needed with additional tamari. If using, mix in the red chili paste and green onions. Toss and serve.

MEXICAN LENTIL SOUP

Serves 4

Energy 190 kcal | Protein 12g | Fat 1g | Net Carbs 25g | P:E Ratio 1:2

Ingredients:

- 2 cups green lentils, rinsed and picked over
- 8 oz diced green chiles
- 5 cups vegetable broth
- 2 cups diced tomatoes and the juices
- 1/2 yellow onion, diced
- 2 celery stalks, diced
- 1 red bell pepper, diced
- 3 cloves garlic, minced
- 1 tbsp cumin
- 1/4 tsp smoked paprika
- 1 tsp oregano
- 1 tsp cayenne pepper
- Pinch of sea salt and black pepper
- Fresh cilantro, for garnish

Instructions:

- Heat vegetable broth in a large pot over medium heat. Add onion, celery, and bell pepper. Sauté until beginning to soften, about 5 minutes. Add garlic, cumin, paprika, and oregano and sauté for another minute.
- Add tomatoes, chiles, lentils, and salt. Bring to a simmer. Simmer the soup with the lid tilted until lentils are tender, about 30–40 minutes. Season to taste with salt and pepper.
- Serve Mexican lentil soup topped with fresh cilantro and a few dashes of cayenne.

TERIYAKI TEMPEH

Serves 2

Energy 256 kcal | Protein 25g | Fat 14g | Net Carbs 12.5g | P:E Ratio 1:1

Ingredients:

- 8 oz tempeh

Tempeh Marinade

- 3 tbsp vegetable broth
- 1 tbsp gluten-free tamari
- 1/2 tsp garlic powder
- 1/4 tsp onion powder

Teriyaki Sauce

- 4 tbsp gluten-free tamari
- 1 tsp sesame or olive oil
- 1 tsp sriracha (or hot sauce)
- 1 tsp rice wine or apple cider vinegar
- 1/2 tsp garlic powder
- 2 tbsp chopped scallions

Instructions:

- Cut tempeh into triangles or squares and steam in a steamer for 10 minutes.
- Add all ingredients for the marinade into a bowl and whisk together. Place tempeh into a dish and pour marinade over. Marinate for at least 20 minutes.

- Spray pan with olive oil or coconut oil cooking spray. Sear the tempeh for 3–5 minutes on each side.
- Mix teriyaki sauce ingredients in a large bowl. Once tempeh is cooked, add tempeh to teriyaki sauce, covering the tempeh. Take tempeh out of the sauce (leaving the extra sauce in the bowl) and add back to the pan.
- Heat tempeh again for about 30 seconds on each side to heat the sauce on the tempeh.
- Turn off the heat and pour the remaining sauce over the tempeh in the pan. Leave for about a minute for the rest of the sauce to thicken.
- Season with scallions.

VEGAN BREAKFAST BURRITOS

Serves 2

Energy 310 kcal | Protein 24.5g | Fat 15g | Net Carbs 12g | P:E Ratio 1:1

Ingredients:

- 12 ounces extra-firm tofu
- 1 cup nopales (fresh if possible), diced or sliced
- 1/2 cup black beans, rinsed and drained
- 1 tbsp garlic
- 1 tsp ground cumin
- Fresh cilantro leaves, coarsely chopped
- Pinch of sea salt and black pepper
- 4 tbsp low-carb salsa
- 4 keto tortillas (Julian Bakery)

Instructions:

- Sauté the nopales until the liquid evaporates. They should be tender and beginning to brown. Set the nopales to the side.
- Using a potato masher or pastry cutter, break the tofu apart into crumbles. Cook until it begins to brown and the texture resembles ground meat.
- Add the black beans and nopales to the tofu. Season with garlic, cumin, salt, and pepper. Cook an additional 4–5 minutes to let the flavors combine.
- Warm the salsa and tortillas. Wrap the sautéed mixture, warmed salsa, and cilantro in a warm tortilla and serve.

EASY VEGAN CHILI SIN CARNE

Serves 4

Energy 203 kcal | Protein 18g | Fat 5g | Net Carbs 15g | P:E Ratio 1:1

Ingredients:

- 16 oz tofu (extra-firm), chopped
- 1 cup red kidney beans, drained and rinsed
- 1/2 cup split red lentils
- 2 cups tomatoes, chopped
- 3 cloves garlic, minced
- 1/2 red onion, chopped
- 2 celery stalks, finely chopped
- 1 red bell pepper, chopped
- 1 tsp ground cumin
- 1 tsp chili powder
- 1 cup vegetable stock
- Pinch of sea salt and black pepper

To serve

- Cooked cauliflower rice (1/2 cup total)
- Coriander, chopped
- A squeeze of lime juice

Instructions:

- Heat the vegetable stock in a large saucepan. Sauté the garlic, onion, celery, carrots, and peppers on medium heat until softened. Add the cumin, chili powder, salt, and pepper and stir.
- Pour in the chopped tomatoes, kidney beans, lentils, and tofu. Simmer for 25 minutes.
- Serve with some cooked cauliflower rice, fresh coriander, and a squeeze of lime juice.

ZUCCHINI GREEK SALAD

Serves 4

Energy 182 kcal | Protein 10.5g | Fat 11.5g | Net Carbs 6.5g | P:E Ratio 1:1.5

Ingredients:

- 8 cups romaine lettuce
- 1 cup edamame
- 2 medium zucchini, spiralized
- 5 tbsp cherry tomatoes
- 4 oz feta cheese, drained
- Pinch of sea salt

Vinaigrette

- 1 tbsp extra-virgin olive oil
- 1 tbsp red wine vinegar
- 1 tsp Dijon mustard
- 1 small garlic clove, minced
- Pinch of sea salt and black pepper

Instructions:

- Spiralize the zucchini using a spiralizer or a potato peeler.
- Add feta, edamame beans, and cherry tomatoes to a large mixing bowl with zucchini. Toss well and refrigerate until ready to serve.
- Prepare the vinaigrette by whisking all the ingredients in a small bowl.
- When ready to serve, pour the vinaigrette over the salad and toss all the ingredients together until the vinaigrette is evenly spread.

TURMERIC SOUP WITH LENTIL AND EDAMAME

Serves 4

Energy 147 kcal | Protein 8g | Fat 5g | Net Carbs 12g | P:E Ratio 1:2

Ingredients:

- 5 cups vegetable broth
- 1 cup edamame
- 1/2 cup red lentils
- 1/2 cup cauliflower rice
- 1 cup kale, chopped, stems removed

- 1/2 onion, grated (about 1 cup)
- 1 small zucchini, grated (about 1 cup)
- 1 tsp turmeric
- 1/2 tsp cumin
- 1 tbsp olive oil
- Pinch of sea salt and black pepper

Instructions:

- Heat olive oil in a medium-sized pot over medium-high heat. Add the onion and zucchini and cook for 1–2 minutes. Add the salt, pepper, turmeric, and cumin, and cook for 2–3 more minutes.
- Stir in the broth and bring to a boil. Once boiling, add the lentils and simmer over low heat for about 20 minutes or until lentils are cooked through.
- In the last couple of minutes of the soup cooking, add the chopped kale and cauliflower rice and serve immediately.

YOGURT PROTEIN BOWL

Serves 1

Energy 168 kcal | Protein 18.5g | Fat 4.5g | Net Carbs 8g | P:E Ratio 1.5:1

Ingredients:

- 1/2 cup plain (or vanilla) low-fat Greek yogurt (Two Good)
- 1/3 cup unsweetened almond milk
- 1/3 cup frozen mixed berries
- 1 tbsp peanut butter powder (Naked Nutrition)
- 1 tbsp vanilla protein powder

- Topped with blueberries and 1 tbsp chia, flax, or sesame seeds

Instructions:

- Blend yogurt with almond milk, mixed berries, peanut butter powder, and protein powder.
- Scoop into bowl and top with berries and seeds.

GREEN POWER SMOOTHIE

Serves 1

Energy 214 kcal | Protein 25g | Fat 9g | Net Carbs 4.5g | P:E Ratio 2:1

Ingredients:

- 1 scoop vanilla protein powder (1 serving)
- 1 cup organic unsweetened almond milk
- 1 cup organic fresh spinach
- 1 tbsp peanut butter powder (Naked Nutrition)
- 1 tsp chlorella or spirulina powder (or other greens powder)
- 1 tsp hemp hulls or chopped pecans

Instructions:

- Blend all ingredients. Pour into glass and top with hemp hulls or chopped pecans.

ABOUT THE AUTHOR

DR. BRIAN MOWLL is a certified diabetes care and education specialist, a master diabetes educator, and the medical director of SweetLife Diabetes Health Centers. He is the six-time host of the global Diabetes Summit and of the number-one-rated *Mastering Blood Sugar* podcast. He also serves on the board of the Low Carb Diabetes Association.

Dr. Mowll has been helping patients and clients reverse type-2 diabetes and blood-sugar problems through his personalized programs for over twenty years. He speaks regularly at health and diabetes conferences around the world and blogs at DrMowll.com.

Brian has four children and resides in Rehoboth Beach, Delaware.

REFERENCES

CHAPTER 1

1   Temneanu, O. R. et al. "Type-2 diabetes mellitus in children and adolescents: a relatively new clinical problem within pediatric practice." *Journal of Medicine and Life* 9, no. 3 (2016): 235–239.

2   Kao, Kung-Ting, and Matthew A Sabin. "Type-2 diabetes mellitus in children and adolescents." *Australian family physician* 45, no. 6 (2016): 401–6.

3   "Cardiovascular Disease and Diabetes." *www.heart.org*. August 20, 2013. www.heart.org/en/health-topics/diabetes/why-diabetes-matters/cardiovascular-disease--diabetes.

4   Brannick, Ben, and Sam Dagogo-Jack. "Prediabetes and Cardiovascular Disease: Pathophysiology and Interventions for Prevention and Risk Reduction." *Endocrinology and Metabolism Clinics of North America* 47, no.1 (2018): 33–50. doi:10.1016/j.ecl.2017.10.001.

5   Kaur, Sharonjeet et al. "Painful diabetic neuropathy: an update." *Annals of Neurosciences* 18, no.4 (2011): 168–75. doi:10.5214/ans.0972-7531.1118409.

6   Vinik, Aaron I. et al. "Diabetic autonomic neuropathy." *Diabetes Care* vol. 26,5 (2003): 1553–1579. doi:10.2337/diacare.26.5.1553.

7   Alicic, Radica Z et al. "Diabetic Kidney Disease: Challenges, Progress, and Possibilities." *Clinical journal of the American Society of Nephrology : CJASN* 12, no. 12 (2017): 2032–2045. doi:10.2215/CJN.11491116.

8   U.S. Department of Health and Human Services. "Diabetic Eye Disease." *National Institute of Diabetes and Digestive and Kidney Diseases*. May 1, 2017. www.niddk.nih.gov/health-information/diabetes/overview/preventing-problems/diabetic-eye-disease.

9   "Diabetes." *Mayo Clinic*. Mayo Foundation for Medical Education and Research. August 8, 2018. www.mayoclinic.org/diseases-conditions/diabetes/symptoms-causes/syc-20371444.

CHAPTER 2

10 Vecchio, Ignazio, et al. "The Discovery of Insulin: An Important Milestone in the History of Medicine." *Frontiers in Endocrinology* 9 (2018). doi:10.3389/fendo.2018.00613.

11 Ibid.

12 Navale, Archana M, and Archana N Paranjape. "Glucose transporters: physiological and pathological roles." *Biophysical Reviews* 8, no.1 (2016): 5–9. doi:10.1007/s12551-015-0186-.

13 Hotamisligil, G S, et al. "Adipose expression of tumor necrosis factor-alpha: direct role in obesity-linked insulin resistance." *Science* 259, no. 5091 (1993): 87–91. doi:10.1126/science.7678183.

14 Sears, Barry, and Mary Perry. "The role of fatty acids in insulin resistance." *Lipids in Health and Disease* 14, no. 121 (Sep. 2015): 29. doi:10.1186/s12944-015-0123-1.

15 Fung, Jason. "A New Paradigm of Insulin Resistance." *Diet Doctor*, December 17, 2016. dietdoctor.com/new-paradigm-insulin-resistance.

16 Shanik, Michael H, et al. "Insulin resistance and hyperinsulinemia: is hyperinsulinemia the cart or the horse?" *Diabetes Care* 31, Suppl 2 (2008): S262–8. doi:10.2337/dc08-s264

17 Kong, Ling Chun et al. "Insulin resistance and inflammation predict kinetic body weight changes in response to dietary weight loss and maintenance in overweight and obese subjects by using a Bayesian network approach." *The American Journal of Clinical Nutrition* 98, no. 6 (2013): 1385–94. doi:10.3945/ajcn.113.058099

18 Hotamisligil, G S et al. "Adipose expression of tumor necrosis factor-alpha: direct role in obesity-linked insulin resistance." *Science* 259, no. 5091 (1993): 87–91. doi:10.1126/science.7678183; Matulewicz, Natalia, and Monika Karczewska-Kupczewska. "Insulin resistance and chronic inflammation." *Postepy Higieny i Medycyny Doswiadczalnej* 70 (December 20, 2016): 1245–1258; Esser, Nathalie, et al. "Inflammation as a link between obesity, metabolic syndrome and type-2 diabetes." *Diabetes Research and Clinical Practice* 105, no. 2 (2014): 141–50. doi:10.1016/j.diabres.2014.04.006; Shoelson, Steven E., et al. "Inflammation and Insulin Resistance." *The Journal of Clinical Investigation* 116, no. 7 (2006): 1793–801. doi:10.1172/JCI29069.

19 Chen, Li, et al. "Mechanisms Linking Inflammation to Insulin Resistance." *International Journal of Endocrinology* (2015): 508409. doi:10.1155/2015/508409.

20 Pizzorno, Joseph. "Is the Diabetes Epidemic Primarily Due to Toxins?" *Integrative Medicine* 15, no. 4 (2016): 8–17.

21 Taylor, Roy, and Rury R Holman. "Normal weight individuals who develop type-2 diabetes: the personal fat threshold." *Clinical Science* 128, no. 7 (2015): 405–10. doi:10.1042/CS20140553; Taylor, Roy. "Calorie restriction and reversal of type-2 diabetes." *Expert Review of Endocrinology & Metabolism* 11, no. 6 (2016): 521–528. doi:10.1080/17446651.2016.1239525.

22 Górski, Jan. "Ceramide and insulin resistance: how should the issue be approached?" *Diabetes* 61, no. 12 (2012): 3081–3. doi:10.2337/db12-1157; Sokolowska, Emilia, and Agnieszka Blachnio-Zabielska. "The Role of Ceramides in Insulin Resistance." *Frontiers in Endocrinology* 10 (August 21, 2019). doi:10.3389/fendo.2019.00577.

23 Hsieh, Ching-Jung, et al. "The relationship between regional abdominal fat distribution and both insulin resistance and subclinical chronic inflammation in non-diabetic adults." *Diabetology & Metabolic Syndrome* 6 (April 1, 2014). doi:10.1186/1758-5996-6-49; Roberts, Christian K et al. "Metabolic syndrome and insulin resistance: underlying causes and modification by exercise training." *Comprehensive Physiology* 3, no. 1 (2013): 1–58. doi:10.1002/cphy.c110062.

24 Sasakabe, Tae, et al. "Association of decrease in carbohydrate intake with reduction in abdominal fat during 3-month moderate low-carbohydrate diet among non-obese Japanese patients with type-2 diabetes." *Metabolism: Clinical and Experimental* 64, no. 5 (2015): 618–25. doi:10.1016/j.metabol.2015.01.012; Volek, Js, et al. "Comparison of energy-restricted very low-carbohydrate and low-fat diets on weight loss and body composition in overweight men and women." *Nutrition & Metabolism* 1, no. 1 (November 8, 2014). doi:10.1186/1743-7075-1-13; Gower, Barbara A, and Amy M Goss. "A lower-carbohydrate, higher-fat diet reduces abdominal and intermuscular fat and increases insulin sensitivity in adults at risk of type-2 diabetes." *The Journal of Nutrition* 145, no. 1 (2015): 177S–183S. doi:10.3945/jn.114.195065.

25 Slentz, Cris A, et al. "Inactivity, exercise, and visceral fat. STRRIDE: a randomized, controlled study of exercise intensity and amount." *Journal of Applied* 99, no. 4 (2005): 1613–1618. doi:10.1152/japplphysiol.00124.2005.

26 Vighi, G et al. "Allergy and the gastrointestinal system." *Clinical and Experimental Immunology* 153, Suppl 1 (2008): 3–6. doi:10.1111/j.1365-2249.2008.03713.x.

27 Giugliano, Dario et al. "The effects of diet on inflammation: emphasis on the metabolic syndrome." *Journal of the American College of Cardiology* 48, no. 4 (2006): 677–85. doi:10.1016/j.jacc.2006.03.052.

28 Zhu, Fengmei et al. "Anti-inflammatory effects of phytochemicals from fruits, vegetables, and food legumes: A review." *Critical Reviews in Food Science and Nutrition* 58, no. 8 (2018): 1260–1270. doi:10.1080/10408398.2016.1251390; Haß, Ulrike et al. "Anti-Inflammatory Diets and Fatigue." *Nutrients* 11, no. 10 (Septempber 30 2019). doi:10.3390/nu11102315; Maleki, Soheila J, et al. "Anti-inflammatory effects of flavonoids." *Food Chemistry* 299 (2019). doi:10.1016/j.foodchem.2019.125124; Di Lorenzo, Chiara, et al. "Plant food supplements with anti-inflammatory properties: a systematic review (II)." *Critical Reviews in Food Science and Nutrition* 53, no. 5 (2013): 507–16. doi:10.1080/10408398.2012.691916.

29 Geer, Eliza B, et al. "Mechanisms of glucocorticoid-induced insulin resistance: focus on adipose tissue function and lipid metabolism." *Endocrinology and Metabolism Clinics of North America* 43, no. 1 (2014): 75–102. doi:10.1016/j.ecl.2013.10.005.

30 Huntriss, Rosemary, et al. "The interpretation and effect of a low-carbohydrate diet in the management of type-2 diabetes: a systematic review and meta-analysis of randomised controlled trials." *European Journal of Clinical Nutrition* 72, no. 3 (2018): 311–325. doi:10.1038/s41430-017-0019-4.

31 Boden, Guenther, et al. "Effect of a low-carbohydrate diet on appetite, blood glucose levels, and insulin resistance in obese patients with type-2 diabetes." *Annals of Internal Medicine* 142, no. 6 (2005): 403–11. doi:10.7326/0003-4819-142-6-200503150-00006.

32 Rothschild, Jeff, et al. "Time-restricted feeding and risk of metabolic disease: a review of human and animal studies." *Nutrition Reviews* 72, no. 5 (2014): 308–18. doi:10.1111/nure.12104.

33 Morais, Jennifer Beatriz Silva, et al. "Effect of magnesium supplementation on insulin resistance in humans: A systematic review." *Nutrition* 38 (2017): 54–60. doi:10.1016/j.nut.2017.01.009.

34 Suksomboon, N, et al. "Systematic review and meta-analysis of the efficacy and safety of chromium supplementation in diabetes." *Journal of Clinical Pharmacy and Therapeutics* 39, no. 3 (2014): 292–306. doi:10.1111/jcpt.12147; Albarracin, Cesar A, et al. "Chromium picolinate and biotin combination improves glucose metabolism in treated, uncontrolled overweight to obese patients with type-2 diabetes." *Diabetes/Metabolism Research and Reviews* 24, no. 1 (2008): 41–51. doi:10.1002/dmrr.755; Singer, Gregory M, and Jeff Geohas. "The effect of chromium picolinate and biotin supplementation on glycemic control in poorly controlled patients with type-2 diabetes mellitus: a placebo-controlled, double-blinded, randomized trial." *Diabetes Technology & Therapeutics* 8, no. 6 (2006): 636–43. doi:10.1089/dia.2006.8.636.

CHAPTER 3

35 Fuhrman, Joel. *The End of Diabetes: the Eat to Live Plan to Prevent and Reverse Diabetes.* New York: HarperOne, 2013.

36 Kendall, Marty. "What Is Nutrient Density?" *Optimising Nutrition.* January 13, 2019. optimisingnutrition.com/nutrient-density-101/.

37 Ibid.

38 Simpson, S J, and D Raubenheimer. "Obesity: the protein leverage hypothesis." *Obesity Reviews: an Official Journal of the International Association for the Study of Obesity* 6, no. 2 (2005): 133–42. doi:10.1111/j.1467-789X.2005.00178.x; Raubenheimer, David, and Stephen J Simpson. "Protein Leverage: Theoretical Foundations and Ten Points of Clarification." *Obesity* 27, no. 8 (2019): 1225–1238. doi:10.1002/oby.22531.

39 Bilsborough, Shane, and Neil Mann. "A review of issues of dietary protein intake in humans." *International Journal of Sport Nutrition and Exercise Metabolism* 16, no. 2 (2006): 129–52. doi:10.1123/ijsnem.16.2.129.

40 Lowe, Michael R., and Meghan L. Butryn. "Hedonic hunger: a new dimension of appetite?" *Physiology & Behavior* 91, no. 4 (2007): 432–9. doi:10.1016/j.physbeh.2007.04.006.

41 Tricomi, Elizabeth, et al. "A specific role for posterior dorsolateral striatum in human habit learning." *The European Journal of Neuroscience* 29, no. 11 (2009): 2225–2232. doi:10.1111/j.1460-9568.2009.06796.x.

42   Avena, Nicole M., et al. "Evidence for sugar addiction: behavioral and neurochemical effects of intermittent, excessive sugar intake." *Neuroscience and Biobehavioral Reviews* 32, no. 1 (2008): 20–39. doi:10.1016/j.neubiorev.2007.04.019.

43   Pursey, Kirrilly M., et al. "The prevalence of food addiction as assessed by the Yale Food Addiction Scale: a systematic review." *Nutrients* 6, no. 10 (October 2014): 4552–4590. doi:10.3390/nu6104552

44   Substance Abuse and Mental Health Services Administration. *Treatment for Stimulant Use Disorders.* U.S. Department of Health and Human Services, Public Health Service. 2014.

45   Gosby, Alison K, et al. "Testing protein leverage in lean humans: a randomised controlled experimental study." *PloS One* 6, no. 10 (2011). doi:10.1371/journal.pone.0025929; Hall, Kevin D, et al. "Ultra-Processed Diets Cause Excess Calorie Intake and Weight Gain: An Inpatient Randomized Controlled Trial of Ad Libitum Food Intake." *Cell Metabolism* 30, no. 1 (2019): 67–77. doi:10.1016/j.cmet.2019.05.008.

46   Naiman, Ted. "About P:E Ratio." Burn Fat Not Sugar. Last modified 2019. www. burnfatnotsugar.com/p2e/AboutP2E.html.

47   Fulgoni, Victor L. 3rd. "Current protein intake in America: analysis of the National Health and Nutrition Examination Survey, 2003-2004." *The American Journal of Clinical Nutrition* 87, no. 5 (2008): 1554S–1557S. doi:10.1093/ajcn/87.5.1554S.

48   Foley, Cian. *Don't Eat for Winter: Unlock Nature's Secret to Reveal Your True Body.* Waterford: UpTheDeise Enterprises, 2017.

49   Villegas, R., et al. "Energy balance and type-2 diabetes: a report from the Shanghai Women's Health Study." *Nutrition, Metabolism, and Cardiovascular Diseases: NMCD* 19, no. 3 (2009): 190–197. doi:10.1016/j.numecd.2008.06.003; Schwartz, Michael W., et al. "Is the energy homeostasis system inherently biased toward weight gain?" *Diabetes* 52, no. 2 (2003): 232–238. doi:10.2337/diabetes.52.2.232.

CHAPTER 4

50   Crew, Bec. "New Study Reveals 84% of Vegetarians Return to Meat." *ScienceAlert*. December 11, 2014. www.sciencealert.com/new-study-reveals-84-of-vegetarians-return-to-meat.

51   Yazıcı, Dilek, and Havva Sezer. "Insulin Resistance, Obesity and Lipotoxicity." *Advances in Experimental Medicine and Biology* 960 (2017): 277–304. doi:10.1007/978-3-319-48382-5_12; Brøns, Charlotte, and Allan Vaag. "Skeletal muscle lipotoxicity in insulin resistance and type-2 diabetes." *The Journal of Physiology* 587, Pt 16 (2009): 3977–3978. doi:10.1113/jphysiol.2009.177758.

52   Kendall, Marty. "Protein weight loss: How Much Do You Need and Why It Works." *Optimising Nutrition*. October 19, 2019. optimisingnutrition.com/ how-does-protein-suppress-your-appetite/.

53   Gosby, A. K., et al. "Protein leverage and energy intake." *Obesity Reviews* 15, no. 3 (March 2014): 183-91. doi:10.1111/obr.12131.

54   Bekelman, Traci A., et al. "Using the protein leverage hypothesis to understand socioeconomic variation in obesity." *American Journal of Human Biology* 29, no. 3 (2017). doi:10.1002/ajhb.22953.

55   Naiman, Ted. "Macro Calculator." *Burn Fat Not Sugar.* Last modified 2020. burnfatnotsugar.com/MacroCalc.html.

56   Ravn, Anne-Marie, et al. "Thermic effect of a meal and appetite in adults: an individual participant data meta-analysis of meal-test trials." *Food & Nutrition Research* 57 (2013). doi:10.3402/fnr.v57i0.19676.

57   Holt, S. H., et al. "A satiety index of common foods." *European Journal of Clinical Nutrition* 49, no. 9 (1995): 675–90.

58   Leidy, Heather J., et al. "The effects of consuming frequent, higher protein meals on appetite and satiety during weight loss in overweight/obese men." *Obesity* 19, no. 4 (2011): 818–824. doi:10.1038/oby.2010.203.

59   Weigle, David S., et al. "A high-protein diet induces sustained reductions in appetite, ad libitum caloric intake, and body weight despite compensatory changes in diurnal plasma leptin and ghrelin concentrations." *The American Journal of Clinical Nutrition* 82, no. 1 (2005): 41–48. doi:10.1093/ajcn.82.1.41.

60   Carbone, John W., and Stefan M. Pasiakos. "Dietary Protein and Muscle Mass: Translating Science to Application and Health Benefit." *Nutrients* 11, no. 5 (May 22 2019). doi:10.3390/nu11051136; Kim, Jung Eun, et al. "Effects of dietary protein intake on body composition changes after weight loss in older adults: a systematic review and meta-analysis." *Nutrition Reviews* 74, no. 3 (2016): 210–224. doi:10.1093/nutrit/nuv065.

61   European Society of Cardiology (ESC). "Crash diets can cause transient deterioration in heart function." *ScienceDaily.* February 2, 2018.

62   Bekelman, Traci A., et al. "Using the protein leverage hypothesis to understand socioeconomic variation in obesity." *American Journal of Human Biology* 29, no. 3 (2017). doi:10.1002/ajhb.22953.

63   Hamdy, Osama, and Edward S. Horton. "Protein content in diabetes nutrition plan." *Current Diabetes Reports* 11, no. 2 (2011): 111–119. doi:10.1007/s11892-010-0171-x.

64   Schoenfeld, Brad Jon, and Alan Albert Aragon. "How much protein can the body use in a single meal for muscle-building? Implications for daily protein distribution." *Journal of the International Society of Sports Nutrition* 15, no. 10 (2018). doi:10.1186/s12970-018-0215-1.

65   Manore, Melinda M. "Exercise and the Institute of Medicine recommendations for nutrition." *Current Sports Medicine Reports* 4, no. 4 (2005): 193–198. doi:10.1097/01.csmr.0000306206.72186.00.

66 Vitale, Kenneth, and Andrew Getzin. "Nutrition and Supplement Update for the Endurance Athlete: Review and Recommendations." *Nutrients* 11, no. 6 (2019). doi:10.3390/nu11061289.

67 Bang, H. O., et al. "The composition of food consumed by Greenland Eskimos." *Acta Medica Scandinavica* 200, no 1-6 (1976): 69–73. doi:10.1111/j.0954-6820.1976.tb08198.x.

68 Delimaris, Ioannis. "Adverse Effects Associated with Protein Intake above the Recommended Dietary Allowance for Adults." *ISRN nutrition* 2013 (2013). doi:10.5402/2013/126929; Luiking, Yvette C., et al. "Regulation of nitric oxide production in health and disease." *Current Opinion in Clinical Nutrition and Metabolic Care* 13, no. 1 (2010): 97–104. doi:10.1097/MCO.0b013e328332f99d.

69 Grimble, George K. "Adverse gastrointestinal effects of arginine and related amino acids." *The Journal of Nutrition* 137, no. 6, Suppl 2 (2007): 1693S–1701S. doi:10.1093/jn/137.6.1693S.

70 Manninen, Anssi H. "High-Protein Weight Loss Diets and Purported Adverse Effects: Where is the Evidence?" *Journal of the International Society of Sports Nutrition* 1, no. 1 (May 2004) 45–51. doi:10.1186/1550-2783-1-1-45.

71 Ko, Gang Jee, et al. "Dietary protein intake and chronic kidney disease." *Current Opinion in Clinical Nutrition and Metabolic Care* 20, no. 1 (2017): 77–85. doi:10.1097/MCO.0000000000000342.

72 Zhang, Yuqing, et al. "Purine-rich foods intake and recurrent gout attacks." *Annals of the Rheumatic Diseases* 71, no. 9 (2012): 1448–1453. doi:10.1136/annrheumdis-2011-201215.

73 Berrazaga, Insaf, et al. "The Role of the Anabolic Properties of Plant- versus Animal-Based Protein Sources in Supporting Muscle Mass Maintenance: A Critical Review." *Nutrients* 11, no. 8 (2019). doi:10.3390/nu11081825.

74 Mangan, P. D. *Muscle up: How Strength Training Beats Obesity, Cancer, and Heart Disease, and Why Everyone Should Do It.* Phalanx Press, 2015.

CHAPTER 5

75 Patterson, Ruth E., et al. "Intermittent Fasting and Human Metabolic Health." *Journal of the Academy of Nutrition and Dietetics* 115, no. 8 (2015): 1203–1212. doi:10.1016/j.jand.2015.02.018.

76 Kerndt, P. R., et al. "Fasting: the history, pathophysiology and complications." *The Western Journal of Medicine* 137, no. 5 (1982): 379–399.

77 Pattillo, Ali. "Is Intermittent Fasting 'Natural'? History Experts React to the Controversy." *Inverse.* July 26, 2019. www.inverse.com/article/57835-intermittent-fasting-evolution.

78 Stewart, W. K. and L. W. Fleming. "Features of a successful therapeutic fast of 382 days' duration." *Postgraduate Medical Journal* 49, no. 569 (1973): 203–209. doi:10.1136/pgmj.49.569.203.

79 Smith, Margaret E., et al. *The Digestive System*. London: Churchill Livingstone, 2010.

80 Lennarz, William J., and M. Daniel Lane. *Encyclopedia of Biological Chemistry*. Amsterdam: Elsevier Academic Press, 2013.

81 Cahill, George F. Jr. "Fuel metabolism in starvation." *Annual Review of Nutrition* 26 (2006): 1–22. doi:10.1146/annurev.nutr.26.061505.111258.

82 Anton, Stephen D., et al. "Flipping the Metabolic Switch: Understanding and Applying the Health Benefits of Fasting." *Obesity* 26, no. 2 (2018): 254–268. doi:10.1002/oby.22065.

83 Heilbronn, Leonie K., et al. "Alternate-day fasting in nonobese subjects: effects on body weight, body composition, and energy metabolism." *The American Journal of Clinical Nutrition* 81, no. 1 (2005): 69–73. doi:10.1093/ajcn/81.1.69; Catenacci, Victoria A., et al. "A randomized pilot study comparing zero-calorie alternate-day fasting to daily caloric restriction in adults with obesity." *Obesity* 24, no. 9 (2016): 1874–1883. doi:10.1002/oby.21581; Stekovic, Slaven, et al. "Alternate Day Fasting Improves Physiological and Molecular Markers of Aging in Healthy, Non-obese Humans." *Cell Metabolism* 30, no. 3 (2019): 462–476. doi:10.1016/j.cmet.2019.07.016.

84 Halberg, Nils, et al. "Effect of intermittent fasting and refeeding on insulin action in healthy men." *Journal of Applied Physiology* 99, no. 6 (2005): 2128–36. doi:10.1152/japplphysiol.00683.2005.

85 Kahleova, Hana, et al. "Eating two larger meals a day (breakfast and lunch) is more effective than six smaller meals in a reduced-energy regimen for patients with type-2 diabetes: a randomised crossover study." *Diabetologia* 57, no. 8 (2014): 1552–60. doi:10.1007/s00125-014-3253-5.

86 Kleitman, N. "Basal metabolism in prolonged fasting in man." *American Journal of Physiology* 77, no. 1 (1926): 33–44. doi:10.1152/ajplegacy.1926.77.1.233; Patterson, Ruth E., et al. "Intermittent Fasting and Human Metabolic Health." *Journal of the Academy of Nutrition and Dietetics* 115, no. 8 (2015): 1203–1212. doi:10.1016/j.jand.2015.02.018.

87 Heilbronn, Leonie K., et al. "Alternate-day fasting in nonobese subjects: effects on body weight, body composition, and energy metabolism." *The American Journal of Clinical Nutrition* 81, no. 1 (2005): 69–73. doi:10.1093/ajcn/81.1.69.

88 Benedict, F. G. *A study of prolonged fasting*. Washington, D.C.: The Carnegie Institute, 1915.

89 Connolly, J., et al. "Selections from current literature: effects of dieting and exercise on resting metabolic rate and implications for weight management." *Family Practice* 16, no. 2 (1999): 196–201. doi:10.1093/fampra/16.2.196; Frey-Hewitt, B., et al. "The effect of weight loss by dieting or exercise on resting metabolic rate in overweight men." *International Journal of Obesity* 14, no. 4 (1990): 327–34.

90 Malinowski, Bartosz, et al. "Intermittent Fasting in Cardiovascular Disorders-An Overview." *Nutrients* 11, no. 3 (2019). doi:10.3390/nu11030673; Carter, Sharayah, et al. "Effect of Intermittent Compared With Continuous Energy Restricted Diet on Glycemic Control in Patients With Type-2 diabetes: A Randomized Noninferiority Trial." *JAMA Network Open* 1, no. 3 (2018). doi:10.1001/jamanetworkopen.2018.0756; Cho, Yongin, et al. "The Effectiveness of Intermittent Fasting to Reduce Body Mass Index and Glucose Metabolism: A Systematic Review and Meta-Analysis." *Journal of Clinical Medicine* 8, no.10 (2019). doi:10.3390/jcm8101645.

91 Lavin, Desiree N., et al. "Fasting induces an anti-inflammatory effect on the neuroimmune system which a high-fat diet prevents." *Obesity* 19, no. 8 (2011): 1586–1594. doi:10.1038/oby.2011.73; Mushtaq, Rubina, et al. "The role of inflammatory markers following Ramadan Fasting." *Pakistan Journal of Medical Sciences* 35, no. 1 (2019): 77–81. doi:10.12669/pjms.35.1.95.

92 Mattson, Mark P., and Ruiqian Wan. "Beneficial effects of intermittent fasting and caloric restriction on the cardiovascular and cerebrovascular systems." *The Journal of Nutritional Biochemistry* 16, no. 3 (2005): 129–37. doi:10.1016/j.jnutbio.2004.12.007; Johnson, James B. et al. "Alternate day calorie restriction improves clinical findings and reduces markers of oxidative stress and inflammation in overweight adults with moderate asthma." *Free Radical Biology & Medicine* 42, no. 5 (2007): 665–74. doi:10.1016/j.freeradbiomed.2006.12.005.

93 Lee, J., et al. "Dietary restriction increases the number of newly generated neural cells, and induces BDNF expression, in the dentate gyrus of rats." *Journal of Molecular Neuroscience* 15, no. 2 (2000): 99–108. doi:10.1385/JMN:15:2:9.

94 Lee, Changhan, et al. "Fasting cycles retard growth of tumors and sensitize a range of cancer cell types to chemotherapy." *Science Translational Medicine* 4, no. 124 (2012). doi:10.1126/scitranslmed.3003293.

95 Safdie, Fernando M., et al. "Fasting and cancer treatment in humans: A case series report." *Aging* 1, no. 12 (2009): 988–1007. doi:10.18632/aging.100114.

96 Ohsumi, Yoshinori. "The Nobel Prize in Physiology or Medicine 2016." *NobelPrize.org.* Nobel Media AB 2020. Accessed August 21, 2020. https://www.nobelprize.org/prizes/medicine/2016/summary/.

97 Bugliani, M., et al. "Modulation of Autophagy Influences the Function and Survival of Human Pancreatic Beta Cells Under Endoplasmic Reticulum Stress Conditions and in Type-2 diabetes." *Frontiers in Endocrinology* 10 (2019). doi:10.3389/fendo.2019.00052.

98 Madeo, Frank, et al. "Essential role for autophagy in life span extension." *The Journal of Clinical Investigation* 125, no. 1 (2015): 85–93. doi:10.1172/JCI73946.

99 Cantó, Carles, and Johan Auwerx. "Calorie restriction: is AMPK a key sensor and effector?." *Physiology* 26, no. 4 (2011): 214–224. doi:10.1152/physiol.00010.2011.

100 Rynders, Corey A., et al. "Effectiveness of Intermittent Fasting and Time-Restricted Feeding Compared to Continuous Energy Restriction for Weight Loss." *Nutrients* 11, no. 10 (2019). doi:10.3390/nu11102442; Pellegrini, M., Cioffi, I., Evangelista, A., et al. "Effects of time-restricted feeding on body weight and metabolism. A systematic review and meta-analysis." *Rev Endocr Metab Disord* 21, (2020) 17–33. doi:10.1007/s11154-019-09524-w.

101 Jamshed, Humaira, et al. "Early Time-Restricted Feeding Improves 24-Hour Glucose Levels and Affects Markers of the Circadian Clock, Aging, and Autophagy in Humans." *Nutrients* 11, no. 6 (2019). doi:10.3390/nu11061234.

102 Mosley, Michael, and Mimi Spencer. *The Fast Diet*. New York: Atria Books, 2015.

103 Trepanowski, John F., et al. "Effect of Alternate-Day Fasting on Weight Loss, Weight Maintenance, and Cardioprotection Among Metabolically Healthy Obese Adults: A Randomized Clinical Trial." *JAMA Internal Medicine* 177, no. 7 (2017): 930–938. doi:10.1001/jamainternmed.2017.0936; Joslin, P. M. N., et al. "Obese mice on a high-fat alternate-day fasting regimen lose weight and improve glucose tolerance." *Journal of Animal Physiology and Animal Nutrition* 101, no. 5 (2017): 1036–1045. doi:10.1111/jpn.12546.

104 Fung, Jason. *The Obesity Code: Unlocking the Secrets of Weight Loss*. Vancouver: Greystone Books, 2016.

105 Wei, Siying, et al. "Intermittent administration of a fasting-mimicking diet intervenes in diabetes progression, restores β cells and reconstructs gut microbiota in mice." *Nutrition & Metabolism* 15 (2018). doi:10.1186/s12986-018-0318-3; Cheng, Chia-Wei, et al. "Fasting-Mimicking Diet Promotes Ngn3-Driven β-Cell Regeneration to Reverse Diabetes." *Cell* 168, no. 5 (2017): 775–788. doi:10.1016/j.cell.2017.01.040.

106 Steven, Sarah, et al. "Very Low-Calorie Diet and 6 Months of Weight Stability in Type-2 diabetes: Pathophysiological Changes in Responders and Nonresponders." *Diabetes Care* 39, no. 5 (2016): 808–815. doi:10.2337/dc15-1942; Taylor, Roy, et al. "Remission of Human Type-2 diabetes Requires Decrease in Liver and Pancreas Fat Content but Is Dependent upon Capacity for β Cell Recovery." *Cell Metabolism* 28, no. 4 (2018): 547–556. doi:10.1016/j.cmet.2018.07.003.

107 Thomas, Dylan D., et al. "Protein sparing therapies in acute illness and obesity: a review of George Blackburn's contributions to nutrition science." *Metabolism: Clinical and Experimental* 79 (2018): 83–96. doi:10.1016/j.metabol.2017.11.020; Bistrian, B. R., et al. "Nitrogen metabolism and insulin requirements in obese diabetic adults on a protein-sparing modified fast." *Diabetes* 25, no. 6 (1976): 494–504. doi:10.2337/diab.25.6.494; Bakhach, Marwan, et al. "The Protein-Sparing Modified Fast Diet: An Effective and Safe Approach to Induce Rapid Weight Loss in Severely Obese Adolescents." *Global Pediatric Health* 3 (2016). doi:10.1177/2333794X15623245; Eneli, Ihuoma, et al. "Using a Revised Protein-Sparing Modified Fast (rPSMF) for Children and Adolescents with Severe Obesity: A Pilot Study." *International Journal of Environmental Research and Public Health* 16, no. 17 (2019). doi:10.3390/ijerph16173061.

108 Chang, Julia, and Sangeeta R Kashyap. "The protein-sparing modified fast for obese patients with type-2 diabetes: what to expect." *Cleveland Clinic Journal of Medicine* 81, no. 9 (2014): 557–65. doi:10.3949/ccjm.81a.13128.

109 Waldbieser, Jill. "8 People Reversed Their Type-2 diabetes Doing This One Thing." *Reader's Digest*. May 20, 2019. www.rd.com/list/how-people-reversed-their-diabetes/.

CHAPTER 6

110 Cahill, G. F. Jr., et al. "Hormone-fuel interrelationships during fasting." *The Journal of Clinical Investigation* 45, no. 11 (1966): 1751–1769. doi:10.1172/JCI105481.

111 Owen, O. E., et al. "Brain metabolism during fasting." *The Journal of Clinical Investigation* 46, no. 10 (1967): 1589–1595. doi:10.1172/JCI105650.

112 VanItallie, Theodore B., and Thomas H. Nufert. "Ketones: metabolism's ugly duckling." *Nutrition Reviews* 61, no. 10 (2003): 327–341. doi:10.1301/nr.2003.oct.327-341.

113 Martini, Luciano. *Encyclopedia of Endocrine Diseases*. Amsterdam: Elsevier Academic Press, 2004.

114 Veech, R. L., et al. "Ketone bodies, potential therapeutic uses." *IUBMB Life* 51, no. 4 (2001): 241–247. doi:10.1080/152165401753311780.

115 Wilder R. M., and M. D. Winter. "The threshold of ketogenesis." *Journal of Biological Chemistry* 52 (1922): 393–401.

116 Kinsman, S. L., et al. "Efficacy of the ketogenic diet for intractable seizure disorders: review of 58 cases." *Epilepsia* 33, no. 6 (1992): 1132–1136. doi:10.1111/j.1528-1157.1992.tb01770.x.

117 Ibid.

118 Puchalska, Patrycja, and Peter A Crawford. "Multi-dimensional Roles of Ketone Bodies in Fuel Metabolism, Signaling, and Therapeutics." *Cell Metabolism* 25, no. 2 (2017): 262–284. doi:10.1016/j.cmet.2016.12.022.

119 Maalouf, Marwan, et al. "The neuroprotective properties of calorie restriction, the ketogenic diet, and ketone bodies." *Brain Research Reviews* 59, no. 2 (2009): 293–315. doi:10.1016/j.brainresrev.2008.09.002.

120 Grandjean, Philippe. "Paracelsus Revisited: The Dose Concept in a Complex World." *Basic & Clinical Pharmacology & Toxicology* 119, no. 2 (2016): 126–32. doi:10.1111/bcpt.12622.

121 Dhatariya, Ketan. "Blood Ketones: Measurement, Interpretation, Limitations, and Utility in the Management of Diabetic Ketoacidosis." *The Review of Diabetic Studies: RDS* 13, no. 4 (2016): 217–225. doi:10.1900/RDS.2016.13.217.

122 Phinney, Stephen, and Jeff Volek. "The Ten Defining Characteristics of a Well-Formulated Ketogenic Diet." *Virta Health.* August 13, 2018. www.virtahealth.com/blog/well-formulated-ketogenic-diet.

123 White, Hayden, and Balasubramanian Venkatesh. "Clinical review: ketones and brain injury." *Critical Care* 15, no. 2 (2011). doi:10.1186/cc10020; Sedej, Simon. "Ketone bodies to the rescue for an aging heart?" *Cardiovascular Research* 114, no. 1 (2018): e1–e2. doi:10.1093/cvr/cvx218; Cotter, David G., et al. "Ketone body metabolism and cardiovascular disease." *American Journal of Physiology—Heart and Circulatory Physiology* 304, no. 8 (2013): H1060–H1076. doi:10.1152/ajpheart.00646.2012.

124 Westman, Eric C. "Is dietary carbohydrate essential for human nutrition?" *The American Journal of Clinical Nutrition* 75, no. 5 (2002): 951–953; author reply 953–954. doi:10.1093/ajcn/75.5.951.

125 Murray, Bob, and Christine Rosenbloom. "Fundamentals of glycogen metabolism for coaches and athletes." *Nutrition Reviews* 76, no. 4 (2018): 243–259. doi:10.1093/nutrit/nuy001.

126 Hue, Louis, and Heinrich Taegtmeyer. "The Randle cycle revisited: a new head for an old hat." *American Journal of Physiology—Endocrinology and Metabolism* 297, no. 3 (2009): E578–E591. doi:10.1152/ajpendo.00093.2009.

127 Manninen, Anssi H. "Very-low-carbohydrate diets and preservation of muscle mass." *Nutrition & Metabolism* 3 (2006). doi:10.1186/1743-7075-3-9.

128 Badman, Michael K., et al. "A very low carbohydrate ketogenic diet improves glucose tolerance in ob/ob mice independently of weight loss." *American Journal of Physiology—Endocrinology and Metabolism* 297, no. 5 (2009): E1197–E1204. doi:10.1152/ajpendo.00357.2009; Pinto, Alessandro, et al. "Anti-Oxidant and Anti-Inflammatory Activity of Ketogenic Diet: New Perspectives for Neuroprotection in Alzheimer's Disease." *Antioxidants* 7, no. 5 (2018). doi:10.3390/antiox7050063; Paoli, A., et al. "Beyond weight loss: a review of the therapeutic uses of very-low-carbohydrate (ketogenic) diets." *European Journal of Clinical Nutrition* 67, no. 8 (2013): 789–796. doi:10.1038/ejcn.2013.116; Harvey, Kristin L., et al. "Ketogenic Diets and Exercise Performance." *Nutrients* 11, no. 10 (2019). doi:10.3390/nu11102296.

129 Hallberg, Sarah J., et al. "Effectiveness and Safety of a Novel Care Model for the Management of Type-2 diabetes at 1 Year: An Open-Label, Non-Randomized, Controlled Study." *Diabetes Therapy: Research, Treatment and Education of Diabetes and Related Disorders* 9, no. 2 (2018): 583–612. doi:10.1007/s13300-018-0373-9.

130 Athinarayanan, Shaminie J., et al. "Long-Term Effects of a Novel Continuous Remote Care Intervention Including Nutritional Ketosis for the Management of Type-2 diabetes: A 2-Year Non-randomized Clinical Trial." *Frontiers in Endocrinology* 10 (2019). doi:10.3389/fendo.2019.00348.

131 Lennerz, Belinda S., et al. "Management of Type-1 Diabetes With a Very Low-Carbohydrate Diet." *Pediatrics* 141, no. 6 (2018). doi:10.1542/peds.2017-3349.

132 Kosinski, Christophe, and François R. Jornayvaz. "Effects of Ketogenic Diets on Cardiovascular Risk Factors: Evidence from Animal and Human Studies." *Nutrients* 9, no. 5 (2017). doi:10.3390/nu9050517; Tan-Shalaby, Jocelyn. "Ketogenic Diets and Cancer: Emerging Evidence." *Federal Practitioner* 34, Suppl 1 (2017): 37S–42S; Włodarek, Dariusz. "Role of Ketogenic Diets in Neurodegenerative Diseases (Alzheimer's Disease and Parkinson's Disease)." *Nutrients* 11, no. 1 (2019). doi:10.3390/nu11010169; Mavropoulos, John C., et al. "The effects of a low-carbohydrate, ketogenic diet on the polycystic ovary syndrome: a pilot study." *Nutrition & Metabolism* 2 (2005). doi:10.1186/1743-7075-2-35.

133 Masood, W., P. Annamaraju, and K. R. Uppaluri. "Ketogenic Diet." *StatPearls* (2021).

134 O'Malley, Trevor, et al. "Nutritional ketone salts increase fat oxidation but impair high-intensity exercise performance in healthy adult males." *Applied Physiology, Nutrition, and Metabolism* 42, no. 10 (2017): 1031–1035. doi:10.1139/apnm-2016-0641.

135 Gajraj, Kim, and Andreas Eenfeldt. "Exogenous Ketone Supplements: Do They Work?" Diet Doctor. November 6, 2020. www.dietdoctor.com/low-carb/keto/exogenous-ketones.

136 Myette-Côté, Étienne, et al. "Prior ingestion of exogenous ketone monoester attenuates the glycaemic response to an oral glucose tolerance test in healthy young individuals." *The Journal of Physiology* 596, no. 8 (2018): 1385–1395. doi:10.1113/JP275709.

137 Cox, Pete J., et al. "Nutritional Ketosis Alters Fuel Preference and Thereby Endurance Performance in Athletes." *Cell Metabolism* 24, no. 2 (2016): 256–68. doi:10.1016/j.cmet.2016.07.010.

138 Hernandez, Abbi R., et al. "A Ketogenic Diet Improves Cognition and Has Biochemical Effects in Prefrontal Cortex That Are Dissociable From Hippocampus." *Frontiers in Aging Neuroscience* 10 (2018). doi:10.3389/fnagi.2018.00391.

139 McKenzie, Amy L., et al. "A Novel Intervention Including Individualized Nutritional Recommendations Reduces Hemoglobin A1c Level, Medication Use, and Weight in Type-2 diabetes." *JMIR Diabetes* 2, no. 1 (2017). doi:10.2196/diabetes.6981.

140 Hallberg, Sarah J., et al. "Effectiveness and Safety of a Novel Care Model for the Management of Type-2 diabetes at 1 Year: An Open-Label, Non-Randomized, Controlled Study." *Diabetes Therapy: Research, Treatment, and Education of Diabetes and Related Disorders* 9, no. 2 (2018): 583–612. doi:10.1007/s13300-018-0373-9.

141 Athinarayanan, Shaminie, J., et al. "Long-Term Effects of a Novel Continuous Remote Care Intervention Including Nutritional Ketosis for the Management of Type-2 diabetes: A 2-Year Non-randomized Clinical Trial." *Frontiers in Endocrinology* 10 (2019). doi:10.3389/fendo.2019.00348.

CHAPTER 7

142 Taylor, R. "Pathogenesis of type-2 diabetes: tracing the reverse route from cure to cause." *Diabetologia* 51, no. 10 (2008): 1781–1789. doi:10.1007/s00125-008-1116-7.

143 Thomas, Dylan D., et al. "Protein sparing therapies in acute illness and obesity: a review of George Blackburn's contributions to nutrition science." *Metabolism: Clinical and Experimental* 79 (2018): 83–96. doi:10.1016/j.metabol.2017.11.020.

144 Palgi, A., et al. "Multidisciplinary treatment of obesity with a protein-sparing modified fast: results in 668 outpatients." *American Journal of Public Health* 75, no. 10 (1985): 1190–1194. doi:10.2105/ajph.75.10.1190.

145 Bistrian, B. R., et al. "Nitrogen metabolism and insulin requirements in obese diabetic adults on a protein-sparing modified fast." *Diabetes* 25, no. 6 (1976): 494–504. doi:10.2337/diab.25.6.494.

146 Pfoh, Elizabeth R., et al. "The Effect of Starting the Protein-Sparing Modified Fast on Weight Change over 5 years." *Journal of General Internal Medicine* 35, no. 3 (2020): 704–710. doi:10.1007/s11606-019-05535-0; Chang, Julia, and Sangeeta R. Kashyap. "The protein-sparing modified fast for obese patients with type-2 diabetes: what to expect." *Cleveland Clinic Journal of Medicine* 81, no. 9 (2014): 557–565. doi:10.3949/ccjm.81a.13128.

147 Lim, E. L., et al. "Reversal of type-2 diabetes: normalisation of beta cell function in association with decreased pancreas and liver triacylglycerol." *Diabetologia* 54, no. 10 (2011): 2506–2514. doi:10.1007/s00125-011-2204-7.

148 Lean, Michael E. J., et al. "Durability of a primary care-led weight-management intervention for remission of type-2 diabetes: 2-year results of the DiRECT open-label, cluster-randomised trial." *The Lancet. Diabetes & Endocrinology* 7, no. 5 (2019): 344–355. doi:10.1016/S2213-8587(19)30068-3.

149 Nackers, Lisa M., et al. "The association between rate of initial weight loss and long-term success in obesity treatment: does slow and steady win the race?" *International Journal of Behavioral Medicine* 17, no. 3 (2010): 161–167. doi:10.1007/s12529-010-9092-y.

150 Astrup, A., and S. Rössner. "Lessons from obesity management programmes: greater initial weight loss improves long-term maintenance." *Obesity Reviews* 1, no. 1 (2000): 17–19. doi:10.1046/j.1467-789x.2000.00004.x.

151 Casazza, Krista, et al. "Myths, presumptions, and facts about obesity." *The New England Journal of Medicine* 368, no. 5 (2013): 446–454. doi:10.1056/NEJMsa1208051.

152 "The Cleveland Clinic Diet's 'PSMF' Approach Results in 50 Pound Weight Loss in Just 80 Days." *Woman's World.* September 5, 2018. www.womansworld.com/posts/diets/cleveland-clinic-diet-psmf-diet-165706.

CHAPTER 8

153 Raatz, Susan K., et al. "Issues of fish consumption for cardiovascular disease risk reduction." *Nutrients* 5, no. 4 (2013): 1081–1097. doi:10.3390/nu5041081; He, Ka, et al. "Accumulated evidence on fish consumption and coronary heart disease mortality: a meta-analysis of cohort studies." *Circulation* 109, no. 22 (2004): 2705–2711. doi:10.1161/01. CIR.0000132503.19410.6B; Tørris, Christine, et al. "Nutrients in Fish and Possible Associations with Cardiovascular Disease Risk Factors in Metabolic Syndrome." *Nutrients* 10, no. 7 (2018). doi:10.3390/nu10070952.

154 Dyall, Simon C. "Long-chain omega-3 fatty acids and the brain: a review of the independent and shared effects of EPA, DPA and DHA." *Frontiers in Aging Neuroscience* 7 (2015). doi:10.3389/fnagi.2015.00052; Hodge W., D. Barnes, and H. M. Schachter, et al. "Effects of Omega-3 Fatty Acids on Eye Health: Summary." *AHRQ Evidence Report Summaries* (2005); Yates, Anthony, et al. "Evaluation of lipid profiles and the use of omega-3 essential Fatty Acid in professional football players." *Sports Health* 1, no. 1 (2009): 21–30. doi:10.1177/1941738108326978; Calder, Philip C. "Omega-3 fatty acids and inflammatory processes." *Nutrients* 2, no. 3 (2010): 355–374. doi:10.3390/nu2030355.

155 Raji, Cyrus A., et al. "Regular fish consumption and age-related brain gray matter loss." *American Journal of Preventive Medicine* 47, no. 4 (2014): 444–451. doi:10.1016/j. amepre.2014.05.037.

156 Yuan, J. M., et al. "Fish and shellfish consumption in relation to death from myocardial infarction among men in Shanghai, China." *American Journal of Epidemiology* 154, no. 9 (2001): 809–816. doi:10.1093/aje/154.9.809.

157 An, Ruopeng, et al. "Impact of Beef and Beef Product Intake on Cognition in Children and Young Adults: A Systematic Review." *Nutrients* 11, no. 8 (2019). doi:10.3390/nu11081797; Hsu, Tsung-Hsien, et al. "Supplementation with Beef Extract Improves Exercise Performance and Reduces Post-Exercise Fatigue Independent of Gut Microbiota." *Nutrients* 10, no. 11 (2018). doi:10.3390/nu10111740

158 "An egg a day could significantly reduce CVD risk." *Cardiovascular Journal of Africa* 29, no. 3 (2018); Qin, Chenxi, et al. "Associations of egg consumption with cardiovascular disease in a cohort study of 0.5 million Chinese adults." *Heart* 104, no. 21 (2018): 1756–1763. doi:10.1136/ heartjnl-2017-312651.

159 Vander Wal, J. S., et al. "Egg breakfast enhances weight loss." *International Journal of Obesity* 32, no. 10 (2008): 1545–1551. doi: 10.1038/ijo.2008.130.

160 Marsset-Baglieri, Agnès, et al. "The satiating effects of eggs or cottage cheese are similar in healthy subjects despite differences in postprandial kinetics." *Appetite* 90 (2015): 136–143. doi:10.1016/j.appet.2015.03.0.

161   Buendia, Justin R., et al. "Long-term yogurt consumption and risk of incident hypertension in adults." *Journal of Hypertension* 36, no. 8 (2018): 1671–1679. doi:10.1097/HJH.0000000000001737; Marin, Ioana A., et al. "Microbiota alteration is associated with the development of stress-induced despair behavior." *Scientific Reports* 7 (2017). doi:10.1038/srep43859.

162   Margolis, Karen L., et al. "A diet high in low-fat dairy products lowers diabetes risk in postmenopausal women." *The Journal of Nutrition* 141, no. 11 (2011): 1969–1974. doi:10.3945/jn.111.143339.

163   Potter, S. M. "Soy protein and cardiovascular disease: the impact of bioactive components in soy." *Nutrition Reviews* 56, no. 8 (1998): 231–235. doi:10.1111/j.1753-4887.1998.tb01754.x; Lichtenstein, A. H. "Soy protein, isoflavones and cardiovascular disease risk." *The Journal of Nutrition* 128, no. 10 (1998): 1589–1592. doi:10.1093/jn/128.10.1589; Bolca, S., et al. "Soy consumption during menopause." *Facts, Views & Vision in ObGyn* 4, no. 1 (2012): 30–37; Yamamoto, Seiichiro, et al. "Soy, isoflavones, and breast cancer risk in Japan." *Journal of the National Cancer Institute* 95, no. 12 (2003): 906–913. doi:10.1093/jnci/95.12.906; Shih, Chao-Ming, et al. "Antiinflammatory and antihyperalgesic activity of C-phycocyanin." *Anesthesia and Analgesia* 108, no. 4 (2009): 1303–1310. doi:10.1213/ane.0b013e318193e919.

164   Shih, Chao-Ming, et al. "Antiinflammatory and antihyperalgesic activity of C-phycocyanin." *Anesthesia and Analgesia* 108, no. 4 (2009): 1303–1310. doi:10.1213/ane.0b013e318193e919.

165   Sears, Margaret E. "Chelation: harnessing and enhancing heavy metal detoxification—a review." *The Scientific World Journal* (2013). doi:10.1155/2013/219840; Otsuki, Takeshi, et al. "Salivary secretory immunoglobulin A secretion increases after 4-weeks ingestion of chlorella-derived multicomponent supplement in humans: a randomized cross over study." *Nutrition Journal* 10 (2011). doi:10.1186/1475-2891-10-91; Mizoguchi, Toru, et al. "Nutrigenomic studies of effects of Chlorella on subjects with high-risk factors for lifestyle-related disease." *Journal of Medicinal Food* 11, no. 3 (2008): 395–404. doi:10.1089/jmf.2006.0180.

166   Olas, Beata. "Berry Phenolic Antioxidants—Implications for Human Health?" *Frontiers in Pharmacology* 9 (2018). doi:10.3389/fphar.2018.00078.

167   Calvano, Aaron, et al. "Dietary berries, insulin resistance and type-2 diabetes: an overview of human feeding trials." *Food & Function* 10, no. 10 (2019): 6227–6243. doi:10.1039/c9fo01426h.

168   Basu, Arpita, et al. "Berries: emerging impact on cardiovascular health." *Nutrition Reviews* 68, no. 3 (2010): 168–177. doi:10.1111/j.1753-4887.2010.00273.x.

169   Fujioka, Ken, et al. "The effects of grapefruit on weight and insulin resistance: relationship to the metabolic syndrome." *Journal of Medicinal Food* 9, no. 1 (2006): 49–54. doi:10.1089/jmf.2006.9.49.

170   Saito, Jun, et al. "The alkalizer citrate reduces serum uric acid levels and improves renal function in hyperuricemic patients treated with the xanthine oxidase inhibitor allopurinol." *Endocrine Research* 35, no. 4 (2010): 145–154. doi:10.3109/07435800.2010.497178.

171 Mahmoud, Ayman M., et al. "Beneficial Effects of Citrus Flavonoids on Cardiovascular and Metabolic Health." *Oxidative Medicine and Cellular Longevity* (2019). doi:10.1155/2019/5484138.

172 Acheson, K J et al. "Caffeine and coffee: their influence on metabolic rate and substrate utilization in normal weight and obese individuals." *The American Journal of Clinical Nutrition* 33, no. 5 (1980): 989–997. doi:10.1093/ajcn/33.5.989; Ruxton, C. H. S. "The impact of caffeine on mood, cognitive function, performance and hydration: a review of benefits and risks." *Nutrition Bulletin* 33, no. 1 (2008): 15–25. doi: 10.1111/j.1467-3010.2007.00665.x.

173 Kwok, Man Ki, et al. "Habitual coffee consumption and risk of type-2 diabetes, ischemic heart disease, depression and Alzheimer's disease: a Mendelian randomization study." *Scientific Reports* 6 (2016). doi:10.1038/srep36500; Wierzejska, Regina. "Can coffee consumption lower the risk of Alzheimer's disease and Parkinson's disease? A literature review." *Archives of Medical Science* 13, no. 3 (2017): 507–514. doi:10.5114/aoms.2016.63599.

174 Casanova, Ester, et al. "Epigallocatechin Gallate Modulates Muscle Homeostasis in Type-2 diabetes and Obesity by Targeting Energetic and Redox Pathways: A Narrative Review." *International Journal of Molecular Sciences* 20, no. 3 (2019). doi:10.3390/ijms20030532.

175 Iso, Hiroyasu, et al. "The relationship between green tea and total caffeine intake and risk for self-reported type-2 diabetes among Japanese adults." *Annals of Internal Medicine* 144, no. 8 (2006): 554–562. doi:10.7326/0003-4819-144-8-200604180-00005.

176 Phinney, Stephen, Jeff Volek, and Brittanie Volk. "How Much Protein Do You Need In Nutritional Ketosis?" *Virta Health*. February 21, 2018. www.virtahealth.com/blog/how-much-protein-on-keto.

177 Chang, Julia, and Sangeeta R Kashyap. "The protein-sparing modified fast for obese patients with type-2 diabetes: what to expect." *Cleveland Clinic Journal of Medicine* 81, no. 9 (2014): 557–565. doi:10.3949/ccjm.81a.13128.

178 Volek, Jeff, et al. *The Art and Science of Low Carbohydrate Living: An Expert Guide to Making the Life-Saving Benefits of Carbohydrate Restriction Sustainable and Enjoyable*. Miami: Beyond Obesity LLC, 2011.

179 Chan, De-Chuan, et al. "Gallbladder contractility and volume characteristics in gallstone dyspepsia." *World Journal of Gastroenterology* 10, no. 5 (2004): 721–724. doi:10.3748/wjg.v10.i5.721.

180 Liu, Ann G., et al. "A healthy approach to dietary fats: understanding the science and taking action to reduce consumer confusion." *Nutrition Journal* 16 (2017). doi:10.1186/s12937-017-0271-4.

CHAPTER 9

181 Bakhach, Marwan, et al. "The Protein-Sparing Modified Fast Diet: An Effective and Safe Approach to Induce Rapid Weight Loss in Severely Obese Adolescents." *Global Pediatric Health* 3 (2016). doi:10.1177/2333794X15623245.

182 Watowicz, Rosanna P., et al. "The Protein-Sparing Modified Fast for Adolescents With Severe Obesity: A Case Series." *ICAN: Infant, Child, & Adolescent Nutrition* 7, no. 5 (2015): 233–241, doi:10.1177/1941406415596342.

183 Thomas, Dylan D., et al. "Protein sparing therapies in acute illness and obesity: a review of George Blackburn's contributions to nutrition science." *Metabolism: Clinical and Experimental* 79 (2018): 83–96. doi:10.1016/j.metabol.2017.11.020.

184 Pfoh, Elizabeth R., et al. "The Effect of Starting the Protein-Sparing Modified Fast on Weight Change over 5 years." *Journal of General Internal Medicine* 35, no. 3 (2020): 704–710. doi:10.1007/s11606-019-05535-0.

185 Institute of Medicine Subcommittee on Military Weight Management. "Factors That Influence Body Weight." *Weight Management: State of the Science and Opportunities for Military Programs.* Washington, D.C.: National Academies Press, 2004.

186 Speakman, John R., et al. "Set points, settling points and some alternative models: theoretical options to understand how genes and environments combine to regulate body adiposity." *Disease Models & Mechanisms* 4, no. 6 (2011): 733–45. doi:10.1242/dmm.008698.

187 Chang, Julia J., et al. "Limited Carbohydrate Refeeding Instruction for Long-Term Weight Maintenance following a Ketogenic, Very-Low-Calorie Meal Plan." *Endocrine Practice* 23, no. 6 (2017): 649–656. doi:10.4158/EP161383.OR.

188 Obeid, O. A., et al. "Refeeding and metabolic syndromes: two sides of the same coin." *Nutrition & Diabetes* 4, no. 6 (2014) doi:10.1038/nutd.2014.21.

189 Pesta, Dominik H., and Varman T. Samuel. "A high-protein diet for reducing body fat: mechanisms and possible caveats." *Nutrition & Metabolism* 11, no. 1 (2014). doi:10.1186/1743-7075-11-53; Leidy, Heather J., et al. "The role of protein in weight loss and maintenance." *The American Journal of Clinical Nutrition* 101, no. 6 (2015): 1320S–1329S. doi:10.3945/ajcn.114.084038; Astrup, A., et al. "The role of higher protein diets in weight control and obesity-related comorbidities." *International Journal of Obesity* 39, no. 5 (2015): 721–726. doi:10.1038/ijo.2014.216; Johnston, Carol S., et al. "Postprandial thermogenesis is increased 100% on a high-protein, low-fat diet versus a high-carbohydrate, low-fat diet in healthy, young women." *Journal of the American College of Nutrition* 21, no. 1 (2002): 55–61. doi:10.1080/07315724.2002.10719194.

190 Soenen, Stijn, and Margriet S. Westerterp-Plantenga. "Proteins and satiety: implications for weight management." *Current Opinion in Clinical Nutrition and Metabolic Care* 11, no. 6 (2008): 747–751. doi:10.1097/MCO.0b013e328311a8c4; Leidy, Heather J., et al. "The role of protein in weight loss and maintenance." *The American Journal of Clinical Nutrition* 101, no. 6 (2015): 1320S–1329S. doi:10.3945/ajcn.114.084038; Schollenberger, Asja E. et al., "Impact of protein supplementation after bariatric surgery: A randomized controlled double-blind pilot study." *Nutrition* 32, no. 2 (2016): 186–192. doi:10.1016/j.nut.2015.08.005; Westerterp-Plantenga, M. S., et al. "High protein intake sustains weight maintenance after body weight loss in humans." *International Journal of Obesity and Related Metabolic Disorders* 28, no. 1 (2004): 57–64. doi:10.1038/sj.ijo.0802461.

CHAPTER 10

191 Kraft J. R., and R. A. Nosal. "Letter: Insulin values and diagnosis of diabetes." *The Lancet* 305, no. 7907 (1975). doi: 10.1016/s0140-6736(75)91922-4.

192 Kraft, Joseph R. *Diabetes Epidemic & You: Should Everyone Be Tested? Absolutely Not! Only Those Concerned about Their Future.* Bloomington: Trafford Publishing, 2008.

193 DiNicolantonio, James J., et al. "Postprandial insulin assay as the earliest biomarker for diagnosing pre-diabetes, type-2 diabetes and increased cardiovascular risk." *Open Heart* 4, no. 2 (2017). doi:10.1136/openhrt-2017-000656.

194 Kraemer, Fredric B., and Henry N. Ginsberg. "Gerald M. Reaven, MD: Demonstration of the central role of insulin resistance in type-2 diabetes and cardiovascular disease." *Diabetes Care* 37, no. 5 (2014): 1178–1181. doi:10.2337/dc13-2668.

195 Price, Catherine. "The Age of Scurvy." *Science History Institute.* August 14, 2017. www.sciencehistory.org/distillations/the-age-of-scurvy.

196 Ibid.

197 Ndrepepa, Gjin, and Adnan Kastrati. "Gamma-glutamyl transferase and cardiovascular disease." *Annals of Translational Medicine* 4, no. 24 (2016): 481. doi:10.21037/atm.2016.12.27; Fentiman, I. S. "Gamma-glutamyl transferase: risk and prognosis of cancer." *British Journal of Cancer* 106, no. 9 (2012): 1467–1468. doi:10.1038/bjc.2012.128; Koenig, Gerald, and Stephanie Seneff. "Gamma-Glutamyltransferase: A Predictive Biomarker of Cellular Antioxidant Inadequacy and Disease Risk." *Disease Markers* 2015 (2015) doi:10.1155/2015/818570.

198 DuBroff, Robert, et al. "Hit or miss: the new cholesterol targets." *BMJ Evidence-Based Medicine* (2020). doi:10.1136/bmjebm-2020-111413; Akyea, Ralph Kwame, et al. "Sub-optimal cholesterol response to initiation of statins and future risk of cardiovascular disease." *Heart* 105, no. 13 (2019): 975–981. doi:10.1136/heartjnl-2018-314253; DuBroff, Robert, and Michel de Lorgeril. "Cholesterol confusion and statin controversy." *World Journal of Cardiology* 7, no. 7 (2015): 404–409. doi:10.4330/wjc.v7.i7.404; Diamond, David M., and Uffe Ravnskov. "How statistical deception created the appearance that statins are safe and effective in primary and secondary prevention of cardiovascular disease." *Expert Review of Clinical Pharmacology* 8, no. 2 (2015): 201–210. doi:10.1586/17512433.2015.1012494.

CHAPTER 11

199 Khawandanah, Jomana and Ihab Tewfik. "Fad Diets: Lifestyle Promises and Health Challenges." *Journal of Field Robotics* 5 (2016): 80.

200 Foxcroft, Louise. *Calories and Corsets: a History of Dieting over Two Thousand Years.* London: Profile Books, 2013.

201 Linn, Robert, and Sandra Lee Stuart. *The Last Chance Diet.* New York: Bantam Book, 1977.

202 Isner, J. M., et al. "Sudden, unexpected death in avid dieters using the liquid-protein-modified-fast diet. Observations in 17 patients and the role of the prolonged QT interval." *Circulation* 60, no. 6 (1979): 1401–1412. doi:10.1161/01.cir.60.6.1401.

203 Palgi, A., et al. "Multidisciplinary treatment of obesity with a protein-sparing modified fast: results in 668 outpatients." *American Journal of Public Health* 75, no. 10 (1985): 1190–1194. doi:10.2105/ajph.75.10.1190; Bistrian, B. R., and M. Sherman. "Results of the treatment of obesity with a protein-sparing modified fast." *International Journal of Obesity* 2, no. 2 (1978): 143–148.

204 Chang, Julia, and Sangeeta R. Kashyap. "The protein-sparing modified fast for obese patients with type-2 diabetes: what to expect." *Cleveland Clinic Journal of Medicine* 81, no. 9 (2014): 557–565. doi:10.3949/ccjm.81a.13128; McDonald, Lyle. *The Rapid Fat Loss Handbook: a Scientific Approach to Crash Dieting.* Salt Lake City: Lyle McDonald Publishing, 2008.

205 Fenech, M. "Recommended dietary allowances (RDAs) for genomic stability." *Mutation Research* 480-481 (2001): 51–54. doi:10.1016/s0027-5107(01)00168-3.

206 Cho, Kyoung Sang, et al. "Recent Advances in Studies on the Therapeutic Potential of Dietary Carotenoids in Neurodegenerative Diseases." *Oxidative Medicine and Cellular Longevity* 2018 (2018). doi:10.1155/2018/4120458; Crowe-White, Kristi M., et al. "Lycopene and cognitive function." *Journal of Nutritional Science* 8 (2019): e20. doi:10.1017/jns.2019.16.

207 Mellen, Philip B., et al. "Effect of muscadine grape seed supplementation on vascular function in subjects with or at risk for cardiovascular disease: a randomized crossover trial." *Journal of the American College of Nutrition* 29, no. 5 (2010): 469–475. doi:10.1080/07315724.2010.10719883.

208 Yoshida, Kazutaka, et al. "Broccoli sprout extract induces detoxification-related gene expression and attenuates acute liver injury." *World Journal of Gastroenterology* 21, no. 35 (2015): 10091–10103. doi:10.3748/wjg.v21.i35.10091.

209 Fu, Zhaozong, et al. "Hesperidin protects against IL-1β-induced inflammation in human osteoarthritis chondrocytes." *Experimental and Therapeutic Medicine* 16, no. 4 (2018): 3721–3727. doi:10.3892/etm.2018.6616.

210 Van Regenmortel, N., et al. "Effect of isotonic versus hypotonic maintenance fluid therapy on urine output, fluid balance, and electrolyte homeostasis: a crossover study in fasting adult volunteers." *British Journal of Anaesthesia* 118, no. 6 (2017): 892–900. doi:10.1093/bja/aex118; Inglott, Anthony S. "Electrolyte Solutions and Body Fluids II. Isotonic Solutions." *Drug Intelligence & Clinical Pharmacy* 6, no. 2 (1972) 69–72. doi:10.1177/106002807200600207.

211 Ghasemi Fard, Samaneh, et al. "How does high DHA fish oil affect health? A systematic review of evidence." *Critical Reviews in Food Science and Nutrition* 59, no. 11 (2019): 1684–1727. doi:10.1080/10408398.2018.1425978; Königs, Anja, and Amanda J. Kiliaan. "Critical appraisal of omega-3 fatty acids in attention-deficit/hyperactivity disorder treatment." *Neuropsychiatric Disease and Treatment* 12 (2016): 1869–1882. doi:10.2147/NDT.S68652; Derbyshire, E. "Do Omega-3/6 Fatty Acids Have a Therapeutic Role in Children and Young People with ADHD?" *Journal of Lipids* 2017 (2017). doi:10.1155/2017/6285218; McGlory, Chris, et al. "The Influence of Omega-3 Fatty Acids on Skeletal Muscle Protein Turnover in Health, Disuse, and Disease." *Frontiers in Nutrition* 6, no. 144 (2019). doi:10.3389/fnut.2019.00144.

212 Innes, Jacqueline K., and Philip C. Calder. "The Differential Effects of Eicosapentaenoic Acid and Docosahexaenoic Acid on Cardiometabolic Risk Factors: A Systematic Review." *International Journal of Molecular Sciences* 19, no. 2 (2018). doi:10.3390/ijms19020532; Chang, Chuchun L., and Richard J. Deckelbaum. "Omega-3 fatty acids: mechanisms underlying 'protective effects' in atherosclerosis." *Current Opinion in Lipidology* 24, no. 4 (2013): 345–350. doi:10.1097/MOL.0b013e3283616364; Moss, Joe W. E., and Dipak P. Ramji. "Nutraceutical therapies for atherosclerosis." *Nature Reviews Cardiology* 13, no. 9 (2016): 513–532. doi:10.1038/nrcardio.2016.103.

213 Gröber, Uwe, et al. "Magnesium in Prevention and Therapy." *Nutrients* 7, no. 9 (2015): 8199–8226. doi:10.3390/nu7095388; Abbasi, Behnood, et al. "The effect of magnesium supplementation on primary insomnia in elderly: A double-blind placebo-controlled clinical trial." *Journal of Research in Medical Sciences* 17, no. 12 (2012): 1161–1169; Mauskop, A., et al. "Intravenous magnesium sulfate rapidly alleviates headaches of various types." *Headache* 36, no. 3 (1996): 154–160. doi:10.1046/j.1526-4610.1996.3603154.x; Garrison, Scott R., et al. "Magnesium for skeletal muscle cramps." *The Cochrane Database of Systematic Reviews* 2012 (2012). doi:10.1002/14651858.CD009402.pub2.

214 Siegel, Jonathan D., and Jack A. Di Palma. "Medical treatment of constipation." *Clinics in Colon and Rectal Surgery* 18, no. 2 (2005): 76–80. doi:10.1055/s-2005-870887.

215 Rao, T. S. Sathyanarayana, et al. "Understanding nutrition, depression and mental illnesses." *Indian Journal of Psychiatry* 50, no. 2 (2008): 77–82. doi:10.4103/0019-5545.42391; Meehan, Meghan, and Sue Penckofer. "The Role of Vitamin D in the Aging Adult." *Journal of Aging and Gerontology* 2, no. 2 (2014): 60–71. doi:10.12974/2309-6128.2014.02.02.1; Penckofer, Sue, et al. "Vitamin D and depression: where is all the sunshine?" *Issues in Mental Health Nursing* 31, no. 6 (2010): 385–93. doi:10.3109/01612840903437657; Foroughi, Mehdi, et al. "The effect of vitamin D supplementation on blood sugar and different indices of insulin resistance in patients with non-alcoholic fatty liver disease (NAFLD)." *Iranian Journal of Nursing and Midwifery Research* 21, no. 1 (2016): 100–104. doi:10.4103/1735-9066.174759.

216 Khosravi, Zahra Sadat, et al. "Effect of Vitamin D Supplementation on Weight Loss, Glycemic Indices, and Lipid Profile in Obese and Overweight Women: A Clinical Trial Study." *International Journal of Preventive Medicine* 9, no. 1 (2018) 63. doi:10.4103/ijpvm. IJPVM_329_15.

CHAPTER 12

217 Bakhach, Marwan, et al. "The Protein-Sparing Modified Fast Diet: An Effective and Safe Approach to Induce Rapid Weight Loss in Severely Obese Adolescents." *Global Pediatric Health* 3 (2016). doi:10.1177/2333794X15623245.

218 Van Gaal, L. F., et al. "Anthropometric and calorimetric evidence for the protein sparing effects of a new protein supplemented low calorie preparation." *The American Journal of Clinical Nutrition* 41, no. 3 (1985): 540–544. doi:10.1093/ajcn/41.3.540.

219 Bakhach, Marwan, et al. "The Protein-Sparing Modified Fast Diet: An Effective and Safe Approach to Induce Rapid Weight Loss in Severely Obese Adolescents." *Global Pediatric Health* 3 (2016). doi:10.1177/2333794X15623245; Pepino, Marta Y., and Christina Bourne. "Non-nutritive sweeteners, energy balance, and glucose homeostasis." *Current Opinion in Clinical Nutrition and Metabolic Care* 14, no. 4 (2011): 391–395. doi:10.1097/MCO.0b013e3283468e7e.

220 Chang, Julia, and Sangeeta R. Kashyap. "The protein-sparing modified fast for obese patients with type-2 diabetes: what to expect." *Cleveland Clinic Journal of Medicine* 81, no. 9 (2014): 557–565. doi:10.3949/ccjm.81a.13128.

221 Harpaz, Dorin, et al. "Measuring Artificial Sweeteners Toxicity Using a Bioluminescent Bacterial Panel." *Molecules* 23, no. 10 (2018). doi:10.3390/molecules23102454.

222 Eneli, I. U., et al. "Rationale and design of a pilot study to evaluate the acceptability and effectiveness of a revised protein sparing modified fast (rPSMF) for severe obesity in a pediatric tertiary care weight management clinic." *Contemporary Clinical Trials Communications* 15 (2019). doi:10.1016/j.conctc.2019.100388.

223 Bhatt, Anjali Amit, et al. "Effect of a Low-Calorie Diet on Restoration of Normoglycemia in Obese subjects with Type-2 diabetes." *Indian Journal of Endocrinology and Metabolism* 21, no. 5 (2017): 776–780. doi:10.4103/ijem.IJEM_206_17; Redman, Leanne M., et al. "Metabolic Slowing and Reduced Oxidative Damage with Sustained Caloric Restriction Support the Rate of Living and Oxidative Damage Theories of Aging." *Cell Metabolism* 27, no. 4 (2018): 805–815. doi:10.1016/j.cmet.2018.02.019; Nicoll, Rachel, and Michael Y. Henein. "Caloric Restriction and Its Effect on Blood Pressure, Heart Rate Variability and Arterial Stiffness and Dilatation: A Review of the Evidence." *International Journal of Molecular Sciences* 19, no. 3 (2018): 751. doi:10.3390/ijms19030751; Purcell, Katrina, et al. "The effect of rate of weight loss on long-term weight management: a randomised controlled trial." *The Lancet—Diabetes & Endocrinology* 2, no. 12 (2014): 954–962. doi:10.1016/S2213-8587(14)70200-1.

224 Bhagavan, N. V., and Chung-Eun Ha. *Essentials of Medical Biochemistry: With Clinical Cases.* Amsterdam: Elsevier Academic Press, 2015; Bistrian, D. R., et al. "Effect of a protein-sparing diet and brief fast on nitrogen metabolism in mildly obese subjects." *The Journal of Laboratory and Clinical Medicine* 89, no. 5 (1977): 1030–1035; Pierro, A., et al. "Characteristics of protein sparing effect of total parenteral nutrition in the surgical infant." *Journal of Pediatric Surgery* 23, no. 6 (1988): 538–542. doi:10.1016/s0022-3468(88)80364-6; Bistrian, B. R. "Clinical use of a protein-sparing modified fast." *JAMA* 240, no. 21 (1978): 2299–2302. doi:10.1001/jama.1978.03290210081040.

225 Simpson, S. J., and D. Raubenheimer. "Obesity: the protein leverage hypothesis." *Obesity Reviews* 6, no. 2 (2005): 133–142. doi:10.1111/j.1467-789X.2005.00178.x.

Made in the USA
Coppell, TX
30 June 2021

58328573R00177